E9-95

C000318551

Sports injuries and their treatment

Sports injuries
and their treatment

illustrated with 142 drawings

John H. C. Colson
FCSP, Dip TP, FSRG, Dip RGRT

William J. Armour
MCSP, Dip TP, FSRG, Dip RGRT

Stanley Paul
London

Copyright © John Colson and William Armour 1961, 1975, 1986

All rights reserved

First published in 1961 by Stanley Paul & Co. Ltd
An imprint of Century Hutchinson Ltd
Brookmount House, 62–65 Chandos Place, Covent Garden,
London WC2N 4NW

Reprinted 1968, 1970
Revised edition 1975
Reprinted 1976, 1979
Second revised edition 1986

Century Hutchinson Publishing Group (Australia) Pty Ltd
16–22 Church Street, Hawthorn, Melbourne, Victoria 3122

Century Hutchinson Group (NZ) Ltd
32–34 View Road, PO Box 40–086, Glenfield, Auckland 10

Century Hutchinson Group (SA) Pty Ltd
PO Box 337, Bergvlei 2012, South Africa

Printed and bound in Great Britain by Anchor Brendon Ltd, Tiptree, Essex

British Library Cataloguing in Publication Data

Colson, John H. C.
    Sports injuries and their treatment.
    Rev. ed.
    1. Sports—Accidents and injuries
    I. Title   II. Armour, William J.
    617.1027   RD97

ISBN 0 09 124180 4

Contents

Preface

When we wrote the first edition of this book over twenty-four years ago we had two aims, and two only, in mind: to produce a guide to the treatment of sports injuries which would be based entirely on our own experiences in clinical practice, and to give practical down-to-earth advice in a concise and readable manner. We were especially anxious to include as much information as possible about strapping and functional support, a somewhat neglected subject in the 1960s.

From its first appearance *Sports Injuries and Their Treatment* was well received by the many therapists and trainers working with injured athletes and players, and we thank them warmly for their continued support and for the many useful suggestions they have made over the years. We have also, of course, had our fair share of criticism – no author can avoid it! Fortunately, most of it has been constructive.

In this completely revised edition of the book we have taken into account the many advances which have been made in recent years in the field of electrotherapy, and have included comprehensive sections on two of the treatments we have found of particular value in the treatment of soft-tissue injuries: interferential therapy and pulsed short-wave therapy. We have also updated and expanded the section on progressive exercise therapy, and made additions to the text concerned with testing for injury.

Looking back on the early days of the book we remember with gratitude the encouragement and advice we received from the late Frederick Pope, MCSP, of Cambridge, an acknowledged expert in the field of sports injuries. We think he would be delighted to know that we continue to follow his very practical guidelines on treatment.

Four of the diagrams in the book (Figs. 41, 48, 49 and 53) were redrawn from illustrations in Pauchet and Dupret's *A Pocket Atlas of Anatomy*, by kind permission of the publishers, the Oxford University Press. We are also indebted to the Football Association for permission to base certain aspects of Chapter 1 on material contained in one of the Association's former publications, *Strapping and Bandaging for Football Injuries*.

Finally, our sincere thanks to Mr Roddy Bloomfield, Director, Stanley Paul and Company, who has not only taken a great personal interest in the book but given us every assistance in preparing this new edition.

John H. C. Colson
William J. Armour

Part 1

Methods of treatment

Chapter 1

General considerations

This chapter gives the background information which is essential for the successful treatment of all types of sports injuries. Section 1 describes the composition of the structures of the body which are commonly injured; Section 2 deals with their reactions to injury; and Section 3 outlines the aims of treatment.

1. Body tissues

Bones and joints

Bones. The bones of the human body form living levers. They are strong and light and constructed to withstand a load of ten or more times the one they are normally called upon to carry. Where speed and efficiency of movement are required the bones are long, with tubular shafts and rounded ends which form the joints; where strength and compactness are necessary, as in the feet and wrists, the bones are short and arranged in groups. When protection of delicate structures is essential the bones are expanded into plates, as in the skull.

Bone is one of the hardest structures of the body, and is made up of two kinds of tissue: an outer dense layer, like ivory, known as *compact* bone, and an inner spongy substance, arranged like a honeycomb, called *cancellous* bone. It is this honeycomb formation which gives strength to the bones, because it forms powerful ties and struts in the areas which carry the main stresses and strains.

The spongy bone contains red marrow, a pulpy substance which is responsible for the manufacture of the red and white blood cells. Another type of marrow, yellow in colour, is found in the shafts of the long bones of the limbs.

Periosteum. The main surfaces of the bones (with the exception of the parts forming joints) are covered by a tough fibrous skin or membrane, the *periosteum*, which carries blood vessels and nerves to the bone. When ligaments or tendons are attached to bones they are blended closely with the periosteum.

Joints. The construction of most of the joints (and this includes those of the limbs) is on the following pattern: (1) The adjacent bone ends are covered by a gristle-like substance, the *articular cartilage*. The cartilage is smooth (which aids movement) and elastic, so that it prevents the bone ends from being damaged by violent blows or jarring movements. (2) A *capsule* or cuff of fibrous inelastic tissue links the bone ends together, and is attached to them close to the margins of the articular cartilage. (3) The capsule is reinforced at certain points by thickened bands of fibres, the *ligaments*. They are tough, inelastic and extremely strong, and are designed to prevent the occurrence of excessive or abnormal movements; on the other hand, they are flexible and pliable, so that they do not obstruct normal movements. (4) A delicate tissue, the *synovial membrane*, lines the joint capsule and covers those parts of the bones which are within the capsule; it ceases, however, at the margins of the articular cartilage. The membrane forms a slippery fluid, known as *synovia*, which spreads over the articular cartilage like a film and acts as a lubricant; it also helps to nourish the cartilage. In appearance this synovial fluid resembles white of egg.

Articular disc. Some of the joints are divided, completely or incompletely, by an *articular disc*, which lies between the bone ends. It is made up of tough fibro-cartilage (fibrous tissue which contains some cartilage cells), and serves to ensure perfect contact between the moving surfaces in any position of the joint; it also helps to spread the lubricating synovial fluid evenly over the joint during movement. The knee joint has two articular discs, the *semilunar cartilages* or *menisci*.

Blood and nerve supply. All the joint structures, with the exception of the articular cartilage and disc, are supplied with blood vessels and nerves. The articular cartilage obtains its nutrition from the network of blood vessels in the synovial membrane, and to some extent from the synovial fluid. It is probable that the articular disc is nourished in the same way.

Muscles, tendons, membranes and skin

Skeletal muscles. The muscles are attached to the bones and form the motor engines of the body. As machines they are unique. There are no man-made mechanical devices with which they can be compared satisfactorily.

Each muscle is composed of numerous bundles of reddish striped fibres which are capable of shortening and lengthening. The bundles are arranged in a parallel manner, and each one is enclosed in an envelope of connective (supporting) tissue. Connective tissue also binds the bundles together, and forms a loose sheath round the entire muscle; in addition, it carries the blood vessels and nerves which supply the fibres.

Muscle fibres are cylindrical in shape, and their stripes are formed by alternating light and dark transverse bands. The length of the fibres varies from about ½ in. in short muscles to more than 12 in. in long muscles.

Muscular contraction. When a muscle contracts a highly organized and intricate telegraph system is brought into action. First the movement to be performed is initiated in a special part of the brain known as the *motor area*; from here movement impulses are transmitted along nerve fibres to 'cell stations' in the spinal cord. Another set of nerve fibres relay the impulses from these cells to the muscle; each nerve fibre divides into anything from 5 to 150 branches, which supply a corresponding number of muscle fibres.

A 'cell station', its nerve fibres and the muscle fibres which it supplies are known as a *motor unit*.

Tendons and aponeuroses. The ends of the muscle are attached to the periosteal coverings of the bones either directly or by means of *tendons* or *aponeuroses*.

Tendons are tough, whitish cords of fibrous tissue; they are often known as 'sinews' or 'leaders'. In muscles which have a wide area of attachment a thin but strong sheet of pearly white fibrous tissue takes the place of the tendon, and this is termed an *aponeurosis*.

Both tendons and aponeuroses are completely inelastic. They are supplied with nerves and a few blood vessels. Some tendons have their own lubricating sheaths of synovial membrane.

Fasciae or protective membranes. The muscles are covered by a strong inelastic membrane, known as the *deep fascia*. In the limbs the fascia is arranged like a close-fitting sleeve, and sends in divisions to separate the various muscles.

The main function of the deep fascia is to assist the muscles when they contract by providing their surfaces with a background of firm pressure. Without this pressure the muscle bellies would bulge outwards on contraction and a great deal of their force would be lost.

Superficial fascia. Immediately above the deep fascia is another protective membrane, the *superficial fascia*. It is made up of a loose-meshed connective tissue which contains fat cells, and is blended with the skin. It facilitates the movements of the skin, and helps to retain the warmth of the body, since fat is a poor conductor of heat; it also serves as a bed for the passage of blood vessels and nerves to the skin.

Skin. The skin consists of two parts – a superficial part, known as the *epidermis*, and a deeper portion, which is called the *dermis*, or true skin. The superficial part consists of several layers of epithelial (protective) cells, which are constantly being replaced as the skin surface is worn away by friction; in this way the underlying true skin, with its blood vessels and nerves, is protected.

Nerves

Nerves are found in all the body tissues. They consist of white cord-like structures, and are made up of a great many nerve fibres which are derived from nerve cells in the brain and spinal cord. The fibres are bound together into bundles by connective tissue, and supplied with blood vessels. The resulting nerve trunk is covered by a thick connective tissue sheath.

Certain nerves are composed entirely of nerve fibres which carry messages to the muscles, causing them to contract, as previously described. Some contain only fibres which are concerned with transmitting messages of sensation (e.g. pain and touch) from the tissues to the brain. Other nerves contain both types of fibres.

Blood and blood vessels

Blood. The total quantity of blood in the body of an averaged-sized man is about nine pints – one-eleventh of the total weight of the body.

The blood consists of a highly complex fluid, the *plasma*, which contains minute blood cells or corpuscles. The plasma is composed of 90 per cent water and 10 per cent solids – protein substances and various salts, especially common salt. The blood cells are of three types, red and white corpuscles, and platelets.

The blood has many functions. Four of the most vital are:

1. To carry oxygen from the air in the lungs to the tissues, and carbon dioxide from the tissues to the lungs;
2. To transport food materials (e.g. glucose and fats) from the stomach and intestines to the tissues;
3. To remove waste products (e.g. urea, uric acid and carbon dioxide) which result when the tissue cells convert to their own use the energy stored in food materials;
4. To assist in the repair of the tissues after injury (*see* p. 17).

Red corpuscles. The red corpuscles are circular disc-shaped cells. They contain a red iron pigment called *haemoglobin*, which not only gives the blood its characteristic colour but is chiefly responsible for the carriage of oxygen and carbon dioxide.

White corpuscles. The white corpuscles, or *leucocytes*, are larger than the red cells and fewer in number. They wander from place to place through the tissues and act as scavengers. After injury, myriads of the cells collect at the site of the damaged structures and engulf or digest the tissue cells which have been destroyed; in this way they facilitate the process of repair. In local infections (e.g. a boil or carbuncle) they remove bacteria and dead white cells in the same way.

Blood platelets. The blood platelets are oval discs, and are much smaller and less numerous than the red cells. They play an important part in the clotting of the blood (p. 16).

Blood vessels. The blood circulates through a closed system of pliable tubes, with the heart as a pump, and supplies practically all the tissues of the body. There are four main types of blood vessels: *arteries, arterioles, capillaries* and *veins*.

Arteries. The arteries carry the blood from the heart to the tissues, and are of various sizes – the largest is a little over an inch in diameter. They are spread over the body and divide and subdivide like the branches and twigs of a tree. Their walls are thick and strong, and are made up of elastic tissue and unstriped muscle.

Arterioles. Each of the small arteries divides into a number of smaller vessels, the arterioles, which are just large enough to be seen by the naked eye. Their walls are composed mainly of unstriped muscle fibres.

Capillaries. The arterioles break up into networks of microscopic vessels called capillaries, which have delicate transparent walls. The diameter of a normal-sized capillary is about $1/3000$ in., and the red blood corpuscles have to pass along it in single file.

Veins. The capillaries gradually increase in size; eventually they form larger vessels, the veins, which return the blood to the heart. The veins are larger and more numerous than the corresponding arteries, but their walls are much thinner. Most veins are provided with valves which open in the direction of the blood flow, and so prevent its reflux.

Lymph and the lymphatics

As the blood flows through the capillaries oxygen and food materials pass through the membranous walls to nourish the tissue cells, while carbon dioxide and other waste products of tissue activity enter the blood in the same way. This exchange is facilitated by the plasma or blood fluid, which 'seeps through the capillary walls and infiltrates the tissues, in much the same way as water from a brook will trickle through a marshy meadow'.[1]

The free blood fluid contains the waste products which are not removed by the capillaries. It is drained away from the tissue spaces by a system of vessels, the *lymphatics*, which at first resemble the capillaries. The smaller vessels join to form larger ones, and ultimately two main trunks are formed; these open into two large veins at the root of the neck. The fluid in the lymphatic vessels is called *lymph*.

---

[1] *The Human Body* (revised ed.). Best and Taylor.

Lymph glands. At certain points along the course of the medium-sized lymph vessels small bean-shaped bodies, known as lymph glands, are found; they act as filters, and prevent any bacteria which enter the lymph current from passing into the blood stream.

The lymph vessels and glands draining any infected area of the body are very liable to become inflamed. The paths of the superficial lymphatics are then often marked out on the skin by painful red lines which lead to swollen, tender glands.

2. Reactions to injury

It is convenient to consider sports injuries in two main groups: (1) Trivial injuries, in which there is no real damage to the tissues, such as strains of muscles and tendons; and (2) More serious injuries, in which there is actual destruction of some of the tissues, such as muscle tears and sprains of ligaments.

Trivial injuries

The reactions of the tissues to trivial injuries are often obscure and difficult to assess; in general they are those of a mild, localized inflamm-ation (p. 17), and pain and stiffness are the main symptoms. Many of the injuries are caused by over-use of the affected part, and clear up with rest; some require support by strapping or bandaging, especially when training is resumed. If more specific treatment is necessary it follows the lines suggested for the more serious injuries.

More serious injuries

Three main changes occur in the tissues when they are more seriously injured: loss of substance or continuity, rupturing of some of the small blood vessels and localized inflammation.

Loss of tissue and rupturing of blood vessels. When some part of a structure is torn or crushed (as by a blow), the small blood vessels of the injured area are ruptured, and bleed into the tissues. The blood seeps between the various tissue layers; its spread is aided by the action of the muscles, the effect of gravity, and the pressure of the membranous coverings. This is the reason why bruising often appears in areas which are some distance from the injured part.

Soon after the injury the capillaries constrict and the blood clots. The blood then consists of a jelly-like substance and a fluid part (the plasma, which has lost certain elements concerned in the clotting process). The clot seals off the ends of the ruptured vessels, and links the torn tissue fibres together. Special connective tissue cells, known as *fibroblasts*, grow into the links and eventually repair the damage.

The fluid part of the escaped blood is drained away by the lymphatics, and eventually returns to the general circulation.

Localized inflammation. At the same time as these changes occur the undamaged capillaries in the neighbourhood of the injury dilate, so that they hold more blood than usual. Their walls become more porous, and a considerable amount of sticky blood fluid (plasma) and a large number of white corpuscles pass through them into the tissues to mingle with the blood from the damaged vessels. The free blood fluid is known as *inflammatory exudate*.

These changes are concerned with repair and healing. The inflammatory exudate stimulates the formation and growth of the fibroblast repair cells. The white corpuscles act as scavengers and remove the tissue cells which have been destroyed; they also deal with the blood clot in the same way.

Signs. The signs of these changes are local heat, redness, swelling and pain. The heat and redness are caused by the extra amount of blood in the arterioles and capillaries of the injured area. The swelling is due partly to the dilation of the capillaries and partly to the accumulation of fluid in the tissues. The pain is either the result of some of the nerves being involved in the injury or of their being compressed by the distended tissues.

Thickenings and adhesions. It is important to restrict the amount of blood and traumatic exudate which escapes into the tissues. Unless this is done the tissues become 'waterlogged', and some of the fibres stick together to form 'gluey' thickenings. If thickenings are allowed to exist they may become organized into fibrous bands, known as *adhesions*. Both thickenings and adhesions limit movement and may cause considerable pain. Old-established adhesions cannot be cleared up by massage, electrotherapy or exercises, as is sometimes thought; they need to be broken down by manipulations performed by the surgeon.

Thickenings and adhesions are particularly likely to occur after injuries when (a) the lymphatic vessels of the injured part have been damaged, so that the tissue drainage system is 'silted up' and disorganized, and (b) the circulation through the sound capillaries of the part is retarded, either because of damage to their arterioles or tension of the tissues; this reduces the number of white blood corpuscles which are available to remove the clot and traumatic exudate. Another, little realized, cause of thickenings and adhesions is the use of vigorous exercise in the early stage of injury. The movements irritate the injured tissues and this leads to the formation of more inflammatory exudate.

Synovial reaction. The reactions previously described also occur when the synovial membranes of joints or tendons are injured; in addition, the undamaged cells of the membranes produce far more fluid than usual, which results in swollen joints and tendons. This change is known as *synovial effusion*; it also occurs if the membranes are irritated rather than actually damaged. *See* p. 148.

Normally the excess fluid is drained away by the lymphatic vessels of the synovial membrane. If the vessels have been damaged or compressed by tissue tension, however, the process is often extremely slow. The continued presence of an abnormal amount of fluid in a joint always causes wasting and loss of power of some of the controlling muscles. *See* Traumatic synovitis of knee, p. 148.

Traumatic effusion. This term is often used to describe the reactions to injury which bring about the accumulation of free fluid in the tissue spaces – inflammatory oozing of blood fluid from sound capillaries, bleeding from torn blood vessels, and (if a synovial membrane has been injured) excessive formation of synovial fluid.

3. Aims underlying treatment

Immediately after the injury, for about 24 to 36 hours

1. *To limit the traumatic effusion (swelling), and so restrict the amount of 'sticky' blood fluid in the tissue spaces.* This is achieved by applying a pressure bandage to the injured part. A calico or crêpe bandage is used over several layers of cotton wool, each layer being compressed by turns of bandage (Fig. 88, p. 127); it is essential that the turns cover the injured part adequately, and extend well above and below it. In general calico bandages are used when treating joints and crêpe bandages when dealing with muscle injuries.

Strapping should not be used to limit traumatic effusion in the early stage of injury; it may produce an uneven, cordlike compression, which may increase the effusion. It should be noted, however, that when an injury does not appear to be of a severe nature, and it is considered essential for the individual to continue to use the injured part, an elastoplast strapping is used instead of a pressure bandage. The principle of allowing an injured player or athlete to resume activity immediately after an injury is basically unsound (*see* Aim 2), and should not be accepted by the trainer or therapist unless he is acting on medical advice.

Ice-cold water. When pressure has been applied the injured part may be immersed in ice-cold water for about 10 to 20 minutes (*see* Fig. 1, p. 24); if immersion is not practicable the bandage may be soaked, the water being applied with a sponge for the same length of time. The wet bandage is then removed, and a new pressure bandage applied.

The cold water relieves pain, and may help to check effusion by causing a local constriction of the capillaries. *See* Cold applications, p. 23.

Local injections of hyaluronidase. In recent years many doctors have used local injections of hyaluronidase (e.g. Hyalase and Rondase) to accelerate the dispersal of traumatic effusion. The injections are used in conjunction with the other forms of physical treatment mentioned in this section.

2. *To prevent movements which might stretch or strain the injured structures and so (a) cause a recurrence of the bleeding, or (b) pull the ends of the torn fibres apart and so hinder repair.* This aim is accomplished by supporting the damaged structures with the pressure bandage in such a way that they are completely relaxed (*see* p. 113), and then resting the injured part. The type of rest required will depend on the severity of the injury; in injuries of the lower limb it may vary from complete rest in bed with the limb raised on pillows (to assist circulation and aid drainage of inflammatory exudate) to semi-rest, e.g. walking with crutches without taking weight on the injured limb. In injuries of the upper limb a triangular sling may be used to provide rest.

3. *To relieve pain.* To a certain extent this aim is achieved by the measures which are taken to fulfil the previous aims – pressure, support, cold applications and rest. In addition some type of pain-relieving drug (e.g. aspirin) may be prescribed by the doctor.

It should be noted that when rest in bed is required for an injury of the lower limb a considerable amount of discomfort and pain is often experienced if the bedclothes are allowed to rest on the limb. A bedclothes support should be improvised by putting a large cardboard box or a pile of books on the mattress at the foot of the bed.

24 to 36 hours after injury, until injured part can be used almost normally

1. *To disperse the traumatic effusion, i.e. (a) to spread the free blood fluid into the surrounding tissues, so that it will be drained away by the uninjured lymphatic vessels and veins, and (b) to assist the drainage of any excess amount of synovial fluid* (p. 18). This aim is accomplished by the use of strapping and various forms of physiotherapy.

Strapping. The injured part is strapped firmly and the player encouraged to use it as normally as possible; in injuries of the lower limb this usually includes walking. The pressure of the strapping on the moving muscles and joints acts as a most efficient form of auto-massage, which improves the circulation and the lymphatic drainage of the part. To increase the effect of the massage the strapping may be applied over a pad of adhesive felt, which is positioned over the injured tissues. *See* Fig. 70, p. 118.

Two types of strapping may be used: (*a*) zinc oxide adhesive plaster (Fig. 107, p. 167), and (*b*) elastoplast combined with supporting strips of zinc oxide plaster (Fig. 106, p. 162). Support is necessary until the traumatic effusion has been completely dispersed; this may take anything from two or three days to two weeks or more, depending on the severity of the original injury.

Protecting the skin. The skin is often sensitive to the adhesive spread, or may be irritated by the strapping being changed frequently, as when daily massage is given. To protect the skin the strapping may be applied *after* the injured part has been covered by a few turns of ordinary cotton bandage, which has been previously soaked in cold water. The strapping must overlap the bottom and top edges of the cotton bandage by about ½ to 1 in., so that it is securely fastened to the skin.

This method of protecting the skin is now superseded by the use of a specialized material known as Underwrap. It consists of a very fine elastic-type fabric which is applied to the injured area before the strapping. The fabric has the property of adhering to itself, but not to the skin.

Joint injuries. In dealing with a joint injury which is associated with a large synovial effusion strapping is not used. A pressure bandage is applied to the joint, the injured limb is rested, and the controlling muscles exercised by static contractions and other *non-weight-bearing* exercises which do not cause movement of the affected joint. *See* Traumatic synovitis of knee, p. 148.

Physiotherapy. Various simple forms of physiotherapy are used to reduce the traumatic effusion, such as contrast baths, massage and exercises. They are usually combined with some form of electrotherapy, such as ultrasound, interferential, standard or pulsed shortwave therapy. The choice depends on the individual preference of the therapist and the precise stage of recovery. The treatments, and their special effects, are described fully in Chapters 2 and 3, pp. 23 and 29.

2. *To prevent movements which might stretch the damaged structures and break down the delicate repair tissue which joins the ends of the torn fibres.* This aim is achieved, as far as possible, by arranging the strapping so that it holds the injured tissues in a relaxed position. *See* Fig. 78, p. 122. With many muscle injuries this is not practicable, and the therapist has to support the affected muscles in a circular manner, as shown in Fig. 106, p. 162, and instruct the player not to put them on the stretch.

3. *To assist repair.* The aim is accomplished by the measures which have been previously outlined for improving the circulation and preventing the damaged structures from being stretched. Some form of heat therapy may also be used to improve the blood supply of the injured part – short-wave diathermy, infra-red radiation, radiant heat or hot packs. These treatments and their special effects are described in Chapter 2, p. 23.

4. *To strengthen the muscles of the affected part, especially those which may have been injured.* The player practises some simple remedial exercises which do not stretch the damaged structures or require too much muscular effort; in practice this means exercising within the limit of pain. 'Strengthening' exercises and the correct exercise technique to employ are described in Chapter 3, p. 29.

5. *To maintain the normal range of movement of the joint or joints of the injured part.* This is done by using exercises of the type suggested above. Unless the joints are exercised their movements may be seriously limited by the formation of thickenings and adhesions. Mobility exercises are described on p. 55.

When the injured part can be used almost normally

1. *To accustom the injured tissues to being without support.* This is achieved by using an elastoplast or crêpe bandage support. Both types of support allow considerable freedom of movement, but provide the injured structures with a certain degree of stability. When elastoplast is used the skin may be protected as described on p. 20.

It is never advisable to take away all support from the injured tissues before they have recovered completely. If this is done the injured part tends to swell when used, owing to a leakage of the blood fluid from the capillaries into the tissue spaces. The swelling gives rise to considerable pain and stiffness.

The leakage of the blood fluid is due to a loss of tone of the capillary walls, which have become accustomed to the firm support of the original strapping.

2. *To disperse any residual effusion or thickenings.* This is accomplished by the auto-massage pressure of the strapping or crêpe bandage, as described in Stage 2. When strapping is used the massage can be localized most effectively by strapping over a pad of adhesive felt. *See* Fig. 70, p. 118. Ultrasonic therapy, remedial exercises and deep massage are also of great value.

3. *To strengthen the muscles of the injured part, and to restore full joint movement.* The player practises all types of strengthening and mobilizing exercises, including weight-resisted exercises. Usually the support bandage or strapping is removed for the treatment session; it may be retained for the stronger exercises.

When training is started

To prepare the injured part for the normal stresses and strains of the game or event. This is done by the player resuming training and carrying out all the normal movements which are expected of him. The injured part should be supported by a firm strapping (*see* p. 20), to prevent a recurrence of the injury.

For two to three months after the injury has recovered fully the player should have the injured part strapped firmly each time he takes part in a game or event. The time factor, of course, will depend on the severity of the original injury.

Chapter 2
Cold, heat and counter-irritation

Cold, heat and counter-irritation have long been recognized as extremely valuable remedies. Often, however, the best results are not obtained from these treatments, mainly because their action on the body is not fully appreciated, and as a consequence their application tends to be confused. For example, heat or counter-irritation is frequently used immediately after an injury instead of cold applications; similarly, cold applications are sometimes used instead of heat treatment in the late stages of injury, and so on.

Cold applications

The simplest and most effective method of applying cold consists of immersing the injured part in ice-cold water. Other methods include ice-packs, compresses and evaporating lotions. Cold applications must be applied immediately, or as soon as possible, after the injury has taken place. It should be noted, however, that cold can be used to relieve pain and associated muscle spasm in the later phases of recovery. Indeed, in recent years many therapists have advocated cold applications for this purpose instead of traditional forms of heat.

Effects of cold. The application of cold to an injured part relieves the pain, through its effect on the nerve endings in the skin: in some cases the relief seems to last for a longer time than when heat is used as a palliative agent. Physiologists investigating the effects of local cooling on the body tissues have found not only that cold reduces the conductivity of nerves, but that the susceptibility of nerves to cooling varies with the type and size of the fibres. Experiments have shown that some smaller diameter fibres are more readily influenced than large diameter fibres.

Work in the USA and this country indicates that if cooling is used solely for the relief of pain temperatures near to freezing point can be used. If the intention is to use cold to reduce muscle spasm and initiate active movement a temperature of between 12°C. and 15°C. (53.6°F. and 59°F.) is best.

Limiting swelling. It is possible that cold applications also help to restrict the traumatic effusion or swelling which accompanies a local inflammation (p. 17), by causing a constriction of the dilated capillaries of the superficial structures. The practical difficulty associated with this form of treatment is that the initial vaso-constriction is followed later by a marked vasodilatation.

Effect on deeper structures. Cold applications have little effect on the capillaries of the deeper structures. This is because the network of blood vessels in the skin acts as an insulator; in other words, the blood flowing through the skin vessels absorbs the cold before it can penetrate to the deeper structures. Because of this, the immediate treatment of soft-tissue injuries should consist of pressure bandaging *combined* with a cold application. *See* Fig. 1.

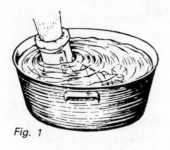

Fig. 1

Immediate treatment of a sprained ankle – pressure bandaging combined with immersion in ice-cold water.

Treatment techniques

Immersion in ice-cold water. This is suitable only for injuries of the wrist, hand, foot and ankle. It consists of immersing the injured part for about 10 to 20 minutes in a pail or deep bowl of cold water to which ice cubes or crushed ice have been added. (Fig. 1). It is advisable to check the temperature of the water with a bath thermometer. After treatment the wet pressure bandage is removed and a new bandage applied.

If immersion is not practicable the pressure bandage may be soaked thoroughly, the water being applied with a sponge.

Wet towels. Several pieces of terry towelling, about 30 × 24 in., are soaked in a mixture of cold water and crushed or flaked ice. The towels are wrung out to get rid of excess moisture, and then applied to the injured area. They are changed every minute, and the whole sequence of cooling should last about 10 to 20 minutes.

From a practical point of view half the number of towels required (having been folded lengthwise) should be left soaking in a bucket while the others are used.

Cold packs. Damp terry towelling bags of a suitable size are filled with flaked or crushed ice. The injured part is wiped with oil to prevent the possibility of an ice burn, and covered with a paper tissue to prevent soiling of the bag. The ice pack is then moulded round the part. If the trunk is being treated it is helpful to hold the pack in place by a broad canvas strap passed round the body.

As an alternative to towelling, plastic or rubber bags may be used.

Reusable packs. Two types of reusable packs are manufactured. They form a very useful substitute for the traditional cold packs, and avoid the inconvenience of melting ice.

Reusable Flexible Ice 'Pax' consist of slim applicators, which store flat in a refrigerator freezer compartment. *3M Cold-Hot Packs* are dual-purpose packs which can be used for cold or hot applications. They are made from a gel which remains flexible between -20 and $+212°$ F. A portion of the water in the gel undergoes a phase change at $32°$ F, which enhances its capacity to cool. The film remains flexible and strong over therapeutic temperature changes, and readily conforms to most body contours.

The Cold-Hot packs are designed to be stored in preconditioning environments (freezer, refrigerator, hot-water bath) and to withstand unlimited cycling of cold to hot conditions. After use the packs should be washed with soap and water or wiped with a disinfectant.

Application. It is best if both types of packs are not applied direct to the skin, but separated from it by a thin layer of towelling.

Ice massage. A paper tissue is wrapped round one end of an ice cube. The cube is then massaged slowly over the painful area for about 5 minutes.

This is a useful form of treatment for relieving pain over a small area (ligaments, for example); it is possible that ice massage acts as a counter-irritant and helps to reduce the conductivity of the pain fibres in the nerves involved.

Cold compresses. A piece of white lint, cut and folded to the required size (to make a double thickness), is soaked in ice-cold water. The lint is squeezed out gently, so that it is not made too dry, and applied to the affected part. It is then covered with a piece of jaconette or oiled silk, and bandaged *lightly* in position with a few turns of cotton bandage. The compress must be changed frequently, and used for about 20 minutes. A pressure bandage is then applied.

In general, cold compresses have a very limited effect.

Evaporating lotions. Useful lotions consist of: (1) diluted methylated spirit (4 ounces of methylated spirit made up to 1 pint with water); (2) lead lotion (strong solution of lead subacetate, 6 minims, methylated spirit, 1 drachm, water to 1 ounce). Diluted lead lotion without spirit, although not a true evaporating lotion, is also used for its pain-relieving properties.

Application. A piece of white lint is soaked in the evaporating lotion and placed on the injured part; it is not covered with oiled silk or jaconette, because this prevents a speedy evaporation of the spirit. The dressing should be used for about 10 to 20 minutes, and kept wet. A pressure bandage is then applied.

Lead lotion is often used in combination with a pressure bandage. One or two strips of white lint are soaked in the lotion and placed over the injured part; the pressure bandage is then applied in the usual way.

Simple forms of heat treatment

The most useful of these treatments consist of: immersion in hot water, hot packs, paraffin-wax baths and electric pads.

Heat therapy must *not be used immediately after an injury, but should be delayed for at least 12 to 24 hours*. It causes a dilatation of the capillaries of the part under treatment, and if used too soon aggravates the inflammatory reaction and encourages bleeding from the torn blood vessels (p. 16).

Effects of heat. The application of heat to an injured part relieves pain and muscle spasm, through its effects on the nerve endings in the skin. This is particularly true of the moist forms of heat, e.g. paraffin-wax and hot packs. Heat also assists in the repair process by increasing the blood supply to the injured area.

Depth of heating

Simple heat treatments have a direct heating effect on the skin. Heating of the structures which lie immediately beneath the skin, such as ligaments, is possible to a *limited* degree by conduction, i.e. the temperature of the skin is raised and the adjacent tissues absorb some of the heat.

Short-wave diathermy, however, is capable of heating the deeper structures, as described in Chapter 3.

Treatment techniques

Immersion in hot water. The heat penetrates the skin to a small degree only, and the heating effect on the deeper tissues is negligible. Generally the treatment is used only when other forms of heat therapy are not available. Immersion time: 20 to 30 minutes.

Hot packs. The heating effect is again superficial. Hot packs are widely used, however, because they form a simple and practical method of applying moist heat in the relief of pain. The towelling pack has now been largely superseded by the 3M Cold-Hot Pack (*see* p. 25) and the Hydropak steam pad. Both packs are relatively inexpensive and can be used at home by the player.

The Hydropak consists of a thick linen pad, 12 by 10 in., which contains a filler which absorbs up to three times its own volume of water. It is stitched into several sections, so that it is flexible and can be moulded to any part of the body.

Technique of use. The pad is placed in a saucepan of hot water and boiled for about 30 minutes. It is then lifted out of the water by the loops which are attached to each corner, and wrapped in four or five thicknesses of Turkish towelling. The pad is then placed on the injured part and covered with two or more layers of towelling to conserve heat. The top towel is usually wound round the area being treated, to hold the pack firmly in place. The pack is left in position for 20 to 30 minutes.

Sheets of foam rubber, ½ in. thick, may be used to replace the towels: this simplifies application. After being boiled, the pad is laid on a piece of foam rubber, 25 × 12½ in., which is folded over it. A towel is placed over the injured part, and covered by another piece of foam rubber, 12½ in. square. The pack is placed on top of the rubber square, and held in place by a towel. The foam rubber can be used a great many times before it needs to be replaced.

Paraffin-wax. When a wax bath is used the heating effect is slightly greater than that produced by the two previous treatments. If the wax is applied as a pack the heating effect is not so pronounced. Wax baths are only suitable for injuries of the hands, wrists, elbows, feet and ankles.

The wax is usually heated to a temperature of between 110°F. and 120°F., and it is best to use a wax with a low melting point (110°F.).

A wax pack is made by using a 2 in. paintbrush, and applying six to eight coats of hot wax to the affected area; the wax may also be applied with a soup ladle. The part is then covered with grease-proof paper, well wrapped in a large piece of old blanket, and left for about 20 to 30 minutes.

Electric pad. Superficial heating only, as with the hot pack. The dry form of heat produced by an electric pad is not so effective in relieving pain as moist heat.

Contrast baths and counter-irritants

Contrast bathing. Alternate hot and cold applications are used to improve the capillary circulation of the superficial tissues. The alternate application of heat and cold causes an alternate dilatation and constriction of the capillary walls, which automatically accelerates the circulation. The treatment must *not be used for at least 12 to 24 hours after injury*.

Techniques. Hot and cold towels are applied alternately to the injured part for a period of about 15 to 20 minutes, each set of towels being kept in contact with the injured part for about 2 minutes at a time. Sprays of hot and cold water may be used instead of towels. In the treatment of foot, ankle, hand and wrist injuries deep bowls or pails of hot and cold water may be used in place of towels or sprays.

Counter-irritants. These are substances which when applied to the body produce a marked dilatation of the skin capillaries and possibly of the capillaries of the deeper structures. The increased blood supply is maintained for 5–8 hours, sometimes more.

Counter-irritants are either used independently or as adjuncts to heat therapy. They must *not be applied during the first 12 to 24 hours after injury*. The most widely used counter-irritants are Scott's dressing and Capsicum ointment.

Scott's dressing. The ointment consists of mercury, camphor, yellow wax and olive oil. The camphor is the chief irritant agent.

The ointment is applied to the smooth surfaces of several strips of white lint, about 2 in. in width. The strips are then arranged on the the injured part (smooth side next to the skin) in a parallel manner, so that the long edge of each strip overlaps the edge of the adjacent strip. A layer of cotton wool is placed over the strips, and the dressing held in place by a crêpe bandage.

The player must be told to remove the dressing if his skin becomes very sore and irritable. Unless this is done blistering may occur.

Capsicum ointment. The ointment contains capsicum oil (the active property of Cayenne pepper), which is extremely irritant to the skin. A small amount of the ointment is rubbed lightly into the skin of the injured part; the residue is then wiped off. A dressing is not necessary.

Chapter 3

Massage and electrotherapy

The physical treatments described here, and in the following chapter, are not used until the early reaction to injury has subsided. The special indications for each form of therapy are outlined in the first chapter of this book under Aims of Treatment (pp. 18–22).

Massage

The chief use of massage in the treatment of injuries lies in its ability to assist the circulation through the veins and lymphatics of the soft structures. The alternate pressure and relaxation effect of the massage manipulations on the tissues acts as a kind of rhythmical pump.

Dispersing traumatic effusion (*see* p. 19). The massage should be started on the sound structures well above the injured part; the best manipulations to use are deep kneading and firm effleurage (stroking in the direction of the heart). After a few minutes the massage should be extended to the upper aspect of the injured area, the pressure being slightly diminished. Gradually the manipulations should encroach on the injured structures, care being taken to avoid producing too much pain in the early stage of recovery. From time to time during the massage session the sound structures above the injured part should be massaged thoroughly.

As the acuteness of the injury subsides the massage should be more confined to the injured area and the adjacent structures; the depth of the manipulations should also be increased. Both transverse and circular frictions are added. Frictions are of great value in dispersing any thickened areas of organized effusion.

Elevation of injured part. In injuries of the limbs the injured part should be elevated on pillows during the massage period, to assist the lymphatic and venous drainage. To achieve an even support it is necessary to pack the pillows under the whole length of the limb.

Assisting in repair process. When massage is used to improve the blood supply of the injured part a similar treatment technique is used, with the exception that elevation is not necessary.

Note. A most comprehensive account of all aspects of massage, including detailed descriptions of the various manipulations used in local and general massage, is given in *Beard's Massage* (3rd edition).[1] The book is essential reading for those who wish to widen their knowledge of this very useful but somewhat neglected form of therapy.

Electrotherapy

Electrotherapy plays an important part in the treatment of sports injuries. The most widely used treatments consist of infra-red radiation, ultrasound, faradism, standard and pulsed short-wave therapy and interferential therapy.

In general, electrical treatments of this type should not be used during the first 24 hours after injury. It is also important that treatment should not be unduly prolonged. Injured sportsmen often attach undue importance to treatment involving the use of impressive-looking electrical apparatus, and attempt to persuade their therapists to continue treatment long after it has ceased to be truly effective. It is bad management, if nothing else, for a player to be receiving short-wave therapy to improve the local circulation when he is capable of a full programme of active exercises.

Infra-red radiation

Two types of apparatus are used for producing infra-red or heat rays: the non-luminous generator, which emits long infra-red rays, and the luminous or radiant-heat lamp, which emits short rays along with visible rays.

Few large-scale radiant-heat lamps are manufactured today (mainly because of the risk of the bulb shattering), but portable radiant-heat cradles or baths, which are placed over some part of the patient, are sometimes used. They usually contain 6 to 12 tungsten-filament bulbs.

Penetration of heat rays and effects. Most of the heat rays are absorbed by the epidermis. Some of the short infra-red rays (from sources of radiant-heat) penetrate to the superficial capillaries of the dermis. The effect is to improve the local circulation.

The long infra-red rays are used in the treatment of skin abrasions,

---

[1] Published by W. B. Saunders Co. (1981), and available in paperback (price £14.95) from Holt-Saunders, Ltd, 1, St Anne's Road, Eastbourne, East Sussex.

ulcers and boils. They have a sedative effect on the sensory nerve endings, and are particularly useful in relieving local pain and reducing protective muscle spasm.

The short infra-red rays are thought to produce heat within the superficial muscles, probably by the process of conduction. This is helpful in the treatment of injuries where an improvement in local circulation is desirable.

Heat of this type must be avoided in the acute phase, however; the local vasodilatation will produce an increase of tissue tension and a marked increase of pain.

Infra-red lasers in physiotherapy

In 1983 infra-red lasers started to be used in the United Kingdom in the treatment of soft-tissue injuries. Basically, the electromagnetic energy released by these lasers stimulates cell metabolism in the area irradiated. This accelerates the interchange of electrolytes through the cell membrane, helping to eliminate waste products and promote healing.

In its simplest form the infra-red laser consists of a pencil-shaped handpiece, which is applied in contact with the skin, perpendicular to the part being treated. It emits pulsed infra-red rays (wavelength: 904 nanometres),[2] with a peak power of over 5 W. A larger type of free-standing laser, operating on the same wavelength and frequency, is also manufactured. It enables the therapist to treat wider areas at one time, and leaves his hands free.

The manufacturers of the apparatus claim that laser treatment will not only produce an analgesic effect after a 3- to 4-minute application, but that this is followed by a noticeable reduction of traumatic effusion. It is also claimed that the infra-red laser has the ability to penetrate tissues to a depth of 3 cm, and so provides a relatively wide treatment range in the field of soft-tissue injuries.

Precautions. During laser treatment special dark glasses must be worn both by patient and operator. Without this protection laser radiation can damage the retina.

Classification of lasers. It should be noted that the infra-red laser has been classified officially as a class 3B laser. The main purpose of classifying laser systems is to avoid confusion between the low- to mid-powered lasers (class 1–3B), and the high-powered surgical lasers (class 4), which require more stringent safety controls.

Advantages and disadvantages. Infra-red lasers have some advantages

---

[2] A nanometre = one thousand-millionth of a metre.

over conventional forms of infra-red radiation (for example, depth of penetration), but these are offset by the very necessary precautions which must be taken when using this form of therapy: use of protective goggles and ensuring the absence of near-by reflective walls and the presence of abundant normal daylight in the treatment room. It is also necessary to have a licence to use laser equipment.

Ultrasonic therapy

Ultrasonic therapy (ultrasound) consists of the use of inaudible sound waves in the treatment of a relatively narrow range of conditions. The sound waves are given off in a beam from the treatment head, or transducer, of the ultrasound generator.

The waves travel in straight lines and gradually diminish in strength as they are absorbed by the tissues through which they pass. As air reflects ultrasound waves, a contact medium, or couplant, must be used between the treatment head and the skin. If the part to be treated can be placed in an arm- or leg-bath, water is the couplant; if direct contact has to be used, the couplant consists of a film of mineral oil spread over the skin of the 'target' area.

Treatment technique. When the injured part is treated in water the treatment head must be kept about 1 or 2 cm away from the skin; the head should be kept moving steadily during treatment, usually in a series of small circles.

Direct contact. When the part is treated by direct contact (and an oil couplant is used) the treatment head must be positioned so that the beam of the ultrasound waves strikes the skin surface at an angle of 90°. As before, the head must be kept moving steadily; this is necessary because the power of the beam is not uniform all over the working surface. It is worth noting that the beam angle need not be perpendicular when an immersion technique in water is used.

Heat is produced in the tissues when the cells are excited by ultrasound waves. If the cells are over-excited they quickly become fatigued and the patient complains of discomfort. The transducer must be moved to another area and the intensity of radiation reduced.

Effects. Over the last 25 years ultrasound has become an accepted part of the treatment of recent soft-tissue injuries. It is worth noting, however, that 'we do not yet know all that happens when living tissues are treated with ultrasound, or even why many of those effects of which we are aware actually occur. This ignorance is, perhaps, excusable, in view of the complexity of the situation. When a target is irradiated with ultrasound, energy is transferred to it by deformation and movement of the material of the target. The more heterogeneous this material is, the more difficult analysis and prediction of the effects of ultrasound upon it become, and a target of living tissue is highly heterogeneous.'[3]

Pulsed ultrasound (which results when the continuity of the ultrasound beam is broken by phased rest periods) has three main effects in the area insonated: the reduction of pain, the absorption of intracellular tissue fluids, and the stimulation of cell activity. It is extremely effective in recent sprains, strains and haematomata.

Contra-indications. Ultrasound is contra-indicated in conditions where the vibration of cells is considered dangerous: blood clots, sepsis, tumours and tuberculosis.

High-frequency electrical energy – short-wave and pulsed short-wave therapy

High-frequency electrical energy was first used as a form of therapy in the latter part of the nineteenth century, largely through the pioneering efforts of two leading scientists of the times: Jacques d'Arsonval, who worked at the University of Paris, and Nikola Tesla, an Austrian physicist working in the USA.

During the 1920s and 1930s the early techniques were considerably refined and developed, largely through the influence of German physicists and physicians, and extensive use was made first of long-wave diathermy and later of short-wave therapy as a means of producing selective heating of the tissues in injury and disease.

Today, long-wave diathermy, which used currents of moderately high frequency and required the electrodes to be in direct contact with the skin (which had many disadvantages), has been superseded by short-wave therapy. In its turn, short-wave therapy is now giving way to pulsed short-wave therapy (PST), a far cry from the early experimental work of d'Arsonval and Tesla.

Short-wave therapy

Short-wave therapy consists of an oscillating electrical current of extremely high frequency. Standard SWD apparatus makes use of a frequency of 27,120,000 cycles per second or 27.12 megahertz (MHz),[4]

---

[3] Dyson, M., and Pond, J. R., (1973). 'The Effects of Ultrasound on the Circulation', *Physiotherapy*, 9, 284.

[4] Hertz (Hz) = unit of frequency in the SI system, equal to one cycle per second. In the UK electrical frequencies are sometimes expressed in terms of cycles per second, or c.p.s.

the electrical energy employed being delivered in the form of a continuous wave of energy.

Electrical and magnetic fields. The electrical energy sources in the short-wave frequency band employed for therapeutic work contain both an electrical or E field and a magnetic or H field: these two fields are out of phase with one another.

Standard short-wave treatment utilizes the electrical field by means of insulated electrodes arranged at some distance from the skin. Air gaps or insulation prevent the direct passage of the current, but allow the short-wave field (the electrical forces arising from the electrodes) to pass through the tissues. This produces an oscillatory current of the same frequency in the tissues.

The frequency is too great for the current to stimulate motor or sensory nerves, but heat is generated by the current overcoming the resistance of the tissues. The heating effect may be deep or superficial, depending on the type and positioning of the electrodes.

The electrodes may be condensor plates or 'shoes', which are separated from the skin by air gaps (Fig. 2), or flexible rubber-covered

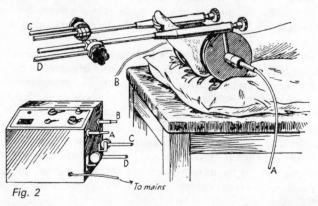

Fig. 2

Deep heating of the ankle joint by short-wave diathermy. The electrode leads (A and B) and the adjustable arms (C and D) have been cut.

electrodes which are separated from the skin by pads of perforated felt.

The electrical or E field is applied by means of condensor or pad electrodes, while the magnetic or H field is applied by means of an inductothermy cable, a long length of plaited wire covered with thick rubber insulation. The cable is either wound round the part to be treated or arranged over the part in the form of a flat helix or 'pancake'; wooden spacers are used to ensure the even spacing of the cable coils. Two or more layers of terry towelling must be used to further insulate the coil from the skin.

Therapeutic effect. The effect of short-wave therapy is to cause a dilatation of blood vessels and an increase of the local blood supply. The
viscosity of the blood is also reduced. This results in better drainage
of the injured part; in turn, this leads to increased absorption and the
dispersal of traumatic inflammation.

Depth of heating. Short-wave therapy does not produce an even heating
of the tissues. The use of condensor or pad electrodes brings about a
greater degree of heating of fat and bone than of muscle tissue. Muscle
heating is best achieved by the use of the inductothermy cable.

Pulsed short-wave therapy

In the last few years pulsed short-wave therapy or PST (also known
as pulsed electro-magnetic energy or PEME) has been widely used in
the treatment of soft-tissue injuries. It has a marked influence on the
reduction of traumatic effusion and the relief of acute and chronic pain.
It is also of particular value in lesions associated with the formation of
excessive connective tissue, e.g. after muscle and tendon tears.

It is interesting to note that PST is also used most successfully in
the treatment of injured animals. The development of portable
machines has opened up this field of work to both horse and
greyhound trainers and veterinary surgeons. For example, one light-
weight model in the Magnetopulse range weighs only 4.98 kilos (11
lbs), while the 'stable' model weighs 10 kilos (22 lbs).

Despite its undeniable value in sports medicine it has taken many
years for pulsed short-wave therapy to be fully accepted as a standard
therapeutic agent in this country, probably because there has been
little authoritative literature published about the exact way in which
its effects are produced. Many therapists are surprised to learn that it
was first introduced into the UK in 1968 after the Mexico Olympic
Games.

Difference between PST and standard SWD. Pulsed short-wave therapy
makes use of the same electrical frequency as standard SWD (27.12
megahertz), but the output of electro-magnetic waves applied (or
pulsed) to the patient is not continuous, but produced for very short
periods at a time, followed by relatively lengthy 'off' periods. Thus
the heating effect is reduced to an absolute minimum. Indeed, in most
instances *heating does not occur in the tissues at all.*

The degree of energy transmitted to the tissues by PST apparatus is
dependent on the pulse width (measured in microseconds, or
millionths of a second), and the number of pulses transmitted in a
second (pulse repetition rate). Writing on this aspect, David E. Oliver,
an engineer with specialized experience of electro-medical equipment,

says: 'With a pulse or burst of energy lasting, say, 65 microseconds (a commonly used pulse duration) there will be about 1,800 complete cycles of HF current before the rest period starts. The rest (or off) period depends on the repetition rate of the pulses and can range between 100 and 800 pulses per second, usually by setting a control on the equipment.

'With a 65 microsecond pulse duration and a repetition rate of, say, 400 pulses per second the off period is 2,435 microseconds. It will be

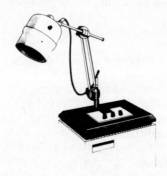

Fig. 3

Pulsed short-wave apparatus (Megapulse) showing drum-shaped electrode. The outer casing of the electrode houses a type of metal coil wound in the form of a flat spiral. When the machine is operating high-frequency currents flow round the coil, which will then produce electromagnetic energy. The EM energy is radiated through the air to the body of the patient positioned close by.

seen that the 'off' to 'on' ratio is some 37 to one. It is this high ratio of periods of rest to that of bursts of energy that is the real technical difference between pulsed short-wave therapy and continuous short-wave diathermy.'[5]

At present, electrotherapy manufacturers use wattage as a rough guide to the energy output of their machines. One experienced physiotherapist who has made a special study of PST considers that therapists need some form of definite measurement on which to base their treatments. He suggests that it would be appropriate to 'use the known quantifiable factors – which are pulse width, pulse repetition rate and, possibly, power settings'.[6]

PST generators. Manufacturers provide a variety of generators. The most widely known are the Megapulse, Diapulse and Therfield. In these generators the applicators are usually either drum-shaped (Fig.

[5] Oliver, D. E. (1984). 'Pulsed Electro-Magnetic Energy – What is it?', *Physiotherapy*, December.

[6] Haynes, C. R. (1984). 'Pulsed High Frequency Energy', *Physiotherapy*, December.

3) or in the form of pads, and provide both electrical and magnetic fields at the same time. Some generators, however, are designed to give either pulsed or continuous short-wave therapy in isolation, e.g. Duffield's ERBE pulsed 2000 Unit.

Physiological effects of PST. Although it is not known with any certainty how pulsed short-wave therapy achieves its therapeutic effects, many therapists believe that it has a direct effect on damaged tissue cells. In an informative article on PST,[7] Christopher Haynes suggests that damaged or injured cells behave in an abnormal manner due to a loss of membrane electrical potential. 'This results in electrochemical changes, particularly an increase in the extra-cellular fluid and swelling which may be responsible for producing pain. Under the influence of the fields produced by PST apparatus, the normal cell potential is restored over a period of around four days, with an accompanying reduction in swelling. This also appears to accelerate wound healing and nerve regeneration.'

Treatment guidelines. PST generators vary in providing different pulse widths and repetition rates. Therapists using the machines need to calculate their own treatment settings, based on both personal experience and the particular type of machine employed.

Certain guidelines need to be followed if the best results from pulsed short-wave therapy are to be achieved.
1. It is essential not to overload the tissues, particularly in the early acute phase of injury. A sensible balance must be achieved between giving too much and too little treatment.
2. An initial treatment time of about 15 minutes is suggested for acute lesions, the PST dosage being kept to a relatively low level.
3. Both treatment time and the degree of electrical energy applied should be gradually increased as the condition improves. Care must be taken not to 'overdose'.

Faradism

Faradism (a low-frequency current) is used to stimulate muscles with an intact nerve supply after injury when the athlete finds it difficult, or impossible, to achieve a normal contraction. When a player sprains the medial ligament of the knee, for example, he may temporarily lose the ability to contract the quadriceps femoris muscle. Pain is the inhibitory factor.

Carefully applied surged faradism can then assist the player to regain control of the muscle. As the quadriceps is stimulated by the current

---

[7] Haynes, C. R. (1985). 'Pulsed Short-Wave Therapy', *Remedial Therapist, 8.*

(Fig. 4) he is asked to try to contract the muscle himself. At first he may find this extremely difficult. Eventually, when the nerve-muscle pathway is re-established, the electrical stimulation should be discontinued.

Faradism can be used very effectively as a form of automassage to reduce swelling within the tissue spaces after injury. The affected part is covered with wet terry towelling (well wrung out); a wet crêpe bandage is then applied to the whole area, and electrodes incorporated at a suitable distance. The muscles are then stimulated for some 20 to 30 minutes with surged faradic current. The contraction of the muscle fibres produces a gentle pressure on the small vessels, which helps to

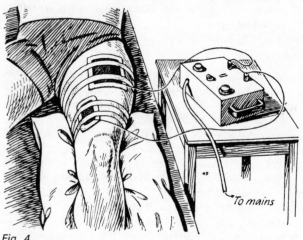

Fig. 4

Faradic stimulation of the quadriceps. The arrangement of the electrodes shown here localizes the current to the vastus medialis and rectus femoris sections of the muscle.

squeeze the blood along the veins and disperse traumatic effusion.

This automassage effect is often combined with elevation of the affected part (pillows or slings being used) to produce a better 'drainage'.

Smart-Bristow induction coil. The original faradic apparatus consisted of the Smart-Bristow induction coil, which was battery-powered and hand-operated. The modern faradic apparatus consists of a small electronic unit: it gives a modified faradic current (50 or so short impulses a second). A surging device, which automatically increases and decreases the strength of the current, is incorporated. Fig. 4 shows surged faradism being used to stimulate the quadriceps femoris muscle, the electrodes being held in place by rubber straps.

Galvanism

Galvanism (a direct electrical current) was once widely used in the treatment of injuries. With the development of short-wave therapy and ultrasound, however, it is now seldom prescribed. This is unfortunate: galvanism has certain specific properties which can be most helpful in certain types of injury.

In general, galvanism produces a marked vasodilatation of the area under treatment; it is therefore helpful in assisting the natural repair processes. The effect is due to marked capillary dilatation, though the exact cause is not fully understood.

The positive electrode is known as the *anode*. It appears to have pain-relieving properties and is useful in the treatment of joint injuries associated with synovial effusion. (Fig. 5.) It is also of considerable value in the early treatment of bruising of the subcutaneous tissues (ecchymosis), such as is seen in 'black eye' and 'cauliflower ear'. The effect of two or three applications of anodal galvanism in dispersing the bruising and relieving the discoloration of the skin is often dramatic.

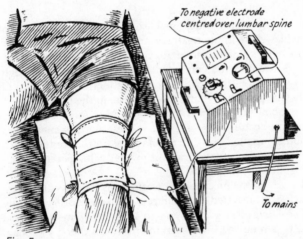

To negative electrode centred over lumbar spine

To mains

Fig. 5

Anodal galvanism being used in the treatment of a synovial effusion of the knee joint. The dotted outline represents the metal plate of the positive electrode. Today an interferential machine may be used to give both galvanic and ionization treatments, *see* p. 44.

The negative electrode or *cathode* has stimulating properties; it is thought to be of use in the treatment of scar tissue in the intermediate phase of injury.

Ionization. The direct current can be used to introduce ionized drugs, such as histamine and sodium salicylate, into the superficial tissues by way of the skin. The amount of drug it is possible to drive through the skin in this manner is obviously extremely limited, particularly when compared with the amount which can be given orally or by injection.

Note. An interferential machine (p. 4) may be used to give galvanic and ionization treatments. Frequencies of 50 to 100 cycles per second are rectified by the machine to give a semi-sinusoidal current with a direct current effect. Application and precautions are the same as for galvanism.

Denervated muscle. When a muscle has an impaired nerve supply, and will not respond to faradic stimulation, the direct current can be used to maintain the activity of the fibres. The muscle bulk is stimulated by an interrupted current, a mechanical interrupter or an electronic unit being used.

Interferential therapy

Interferential therapy is now widely practised in the UK and has been found of particular value in the treatment of soft-tissue injuries. Many therapists think of it as a new form of therapy. In actual fact, interferential therapy was used on the continent in the early 1950s, although only a few physiotherapists in the United Kingdom employed it and appreciated its true potential. Partly this was due to the fact that most of the literature about the treatment was confined to foreign journals. In addition, many doctors were inclined to view the treatment with either suspicion or apathy, particularly as it was introduced at much the same time as powerful new drugs of proven value became available, e.g. cortisone.

Specialized work on the mechanism of pain in the last twenty years, however, which demonstrated that pain could be relieved significantly by the use of selective electrical currents to stimulate primary afferent neurones, led to a renewed interest in interferential therapy. Today, it is recognized as an effective form of therapy, not only in the treatment of recent injuries but in a variety of other conditions, ranging from osteoarthritis and 'frozen' shoulder to acute back pain and intervertebral disc lesions. In stating this, though, it must be emphasized that interferential therapy is by no means a cure-all.

The theory underlying interferential therapy is complex. Basically, two alternating currents of medium frequency are applied to the body in such a way that they cross each other and combine to produce a therapeutic *low-frequency* current at a pre-determined point, e.g. at the central area of a painful joint. (Figs. 6 and 7.) In the past, using standard electrotherapy equipment, it was not possible to introduce low-frequency currents into the body because of the high resistance or impedance of the skin to these currents. Any attempt to achieve this would have resulted in great physical discomfort for the patient. In addition, ulceration at the sites of application of the current would have occurred, due to electrolysis of the tissue fluids.

It should be noted that where two medium-frequency alternating currents cross or intersect in the body the frequency of the resulting current is equal to the difference between the two. For example, if one

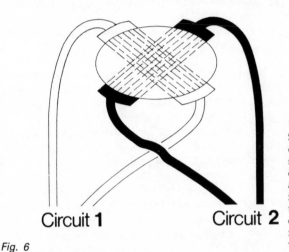

Circuit 1   Circuit 2

Fig. 6

Schematic diagram showing classic application of interferential therapy by four-electrode method. *Cf.* with Fig. 7.

Fig. 6

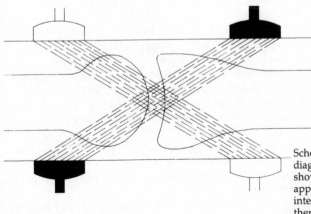

Schematic diagram showing correct application of interferential therapy, so that the two currents cross within the joint.

Fig. 7

current has a frequency of 4,000 cycles per second and the other of 3,900 c.p.s., the resulting current at the intersection has a frequency of 100 cycles per second. Technically, this is referred to as a beat rhythm or interferential field of 0–100 c.p.s.

Application. The medium-frequency currents produced by the inter-ferential machine are applied to the body by means of electrodes of various types. The electrical fields produced in the tissues will depend on the size and position of the electrodes, and great care must be taken over their arrangement.

Two main types of electrodes are used: plate electrodes and vacuum electrodes.

Plate electrodes. In their simplest form plate electrodes may be made of metal. Because metal plates crack easily, manufacturers have intro-duced plates made of conducting rubber. They are easier to position on the body and more comfortable for the patient.

Before use plate electrodes are covered with absorbent material (e.g. Spontex), which is soaked in water or a solution of bicarbonate of soda. Ordinary plastic foam must *not* be used for this purpose; it is not capable of conducting the current.

Plate electrodes are attached to the patient's body by means of straps or crêpe bandages. On the whole, bandages are easier to use and more comfortable for the patient. Unless the electrodes are in firm contact with the skin the patient will not only experience some discomfort during treatment, but will not be able to tolerate as much current.

Vacuum electrodes (Fig. 8). These consist of circular plate electrodes enclosed in rubber suction cups. They are connected to an interferential machine which is capable of producing a vacuum. Each cup is equipped with a piece of Spontex, which lies over the plate component. Before application the sponges are soaked in water or a solution of bicarbonate of soda, and squeezed gently to remove any excess moisture.

The vacuum mechanism of the interferential machine is operated to produce sufficient suction to allow the cups to stay in position on the patient's skin. Too much suction must not be used; it can lead to bruising. On the other hand, too little may allow the cups to be unstable and fall off.

Throughout the treatment the suction must be pulsed at the desired rate, and not maintained at a constant level. This produces a beneficial pulsating massage effect. Most patients find a medium-frequency pulsation the most comfortable.

Vacuum electrodes are said to reduce the resistance of the skin and tissues to medium-frequency currents by increasing the amount of blood and tissue fluid immediately beneath the electrodes.

In practice, it has been found that the most useful frequencies to employ in the treatment of sports injuries are: (a) 90–100 cycles per second; (b) 0–100 c.p.s.; and (c) 0–10 c.p.s.; all given rhythmically.

Frequencies of 90–100 c.p.s. have a beneficial pain-relieving effect; frequencies of 0–100 c.p.s. appear to promote the localized flow of blood and lymph, and assist in dispersing traumatic effusion; while frequencies of 0–10 c.p.s. (which produce local muscular activity) help in dispersing traumatic exudate and in mobilizing early scar tissue. This latter effect is of great importance.

Frequencies of 90–100 c.p.s. and 0–100 c.p.s. are used when there is no likelihood of further bleeding occurring. Each of these frequencies

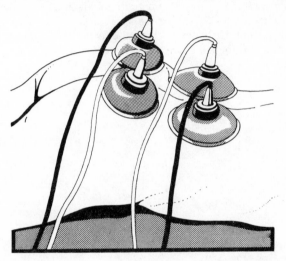

Fig. 8
Interferential therapy: vacuum electrodes being used in the treatment of an injury of the lumbar spine.

can be used up to a maximum of 10 minutes, three or four times a day. After three or four days, if further treatment is necessary, frequencies of 90–100 c.p.s. can be discontinued, and those of 0–10 c.p.s. used.

Duration of treatment. As a general rule the treatment time for interferential therapy is relatively short. An initial treatment may start at 10 to 15 minutes, and be increased to 20 minutes. The total treatment time when one area is being treated should not exceed 30 minutes.

Treatment is usually given daily for a period of about five days. After this, if the condition is improving, treatment is given on alternate days.

Current intensity. In general, the intensity of current employed in an interferential treatment should produce a definite, comfortable prickling sensation, but no muscular contraction.

Interference by short-wave generators. It is important that the interferential unit should not be sited near to a short-wave therapy generator. If the machines are operating at the same time the powerful electrical fields produced by the short-wave generator can have a disruptive effect on the electronic circuits of the interferential unit.

The interferential unit should be sited at a minimum distance of 20 feet from the short-wave generator. Preferably, the two units should be housed in separate rooms.

Direct current effect. An interferential machine is capable of being used to give traditional galvanic and ionization treatments, as described on p. 39. Frequencies of 50–100 c.p.s. are rectified to give a semi-sinusoidal current with direct current effect. Precautions to avoid caustic burns of the skin are necessary, as in ordinary galvanic treatment.

Chapter 4
Progressive exercise therapy

Three main types of specific remedial exercises are used in the treatment of sports injuries: (1) *Strengthening exercises* to redevelop muscles weakened by injury or disuse; (2) *Mobility exercises* to increase the range of movement of joints with restricted function; and (3) *Coordination exercises* to develop physical dexterity and neuromuscular interplay, and so restore the sportsman's confidence in his ability to move freely when following his chosen sport.

For the best results specific exercises must be combined whenever possible with general exercises, so as to coordinate the movements of the injured part with the rest of the body. It is also frequently necessary to combine treatment by exercise with various forms of passive therapy, such as massage and electrotherapy.

Progression. For the therapist who specializes in the treatment of soft-tissue injuries the art of exercise therapy lies not only in choosing the right grades of exercises for the appropriate stages of recovery, but of appreciating the importance of progressing the exercises in a systematic manner. All too often treatment by exercise therapy fails in its objective because the principle of progression is either poorly applied or overlooked.

Strengthening exercises

Strengthening exercises are classified in three groups: (1) Static contractions of the muscles, without joint movement; (2) Free movements of the joints; and (3) Resisted exercises.

Static contractions

Static contractions are used when movement is first allowed after injury. The player attempts to contract the main muscle groups of the injured part without moving the joints. This is easiest to achieve if the muscles are first placed in a short position. For example, to contract the quadriceps femoris muscle on the front of the thigh (Fig. 42, p. 88) the player sits on a massage couch with the legs supported and knees straight. He then attempts to press the back of the knee against the couch. He 'holds' the muscle in the contracted state for a moment or two, and then allows it to return slowly to the resting state. The exercise is repeated with the quadriceps of the other leg; this allows the other muscle to relax, and achieves a balanced interplay between the two muscle groups.

For the best results static contractions should be performed on a 'little and often' basis, and not practised for a set number of times each day.

Free exercises

Free exercises are used in all stages of recovery – with the exception of the period immediately after the injury – and consist of ordinary joint movements and gymnastic exercises. For success the exercises must be progressed smoothly, both in time (number of repetitions) and strength.

Exercise technique. Each exercise should be performed fairly slowly, and with complete control. The movements should be taken to the full extent and 'held' in position for a moment. The player must be trained to relax the acting muscles at the end of each movement; when the arms or legs are moved in turn this occurs in a natural manner.

Some examples of progressive strengthening exercises are given here.[1]

Progressive exercises for calf muscles

Ex. 1. The player takes up a half-lying position (Fig. 61, p. 114) on a massage couch with a pillow arranged under the legs to keep the heels clear of the couch top. He points one foot down as much as possible (Fig. 9), 'holds' the final position for a moment, and then allows the foot to return to its former place. He repeats the exercise with the other foot.

Ex. 2. As the previous exercise, but the player lies facing downwards. (Fig. 10.) The range of movement is larger than in the first exercise.

Ex. 3. The player stands with the feet about 2 in. apart and facing straight forward; he holds the back of a chair or a wall-bar. He raises the heels from the floor as far as possible, using his arms to take some of the body-weight. (Fig. 11.) He 'holds' the final position for a moment

---

[1] Full lists of progressive exercises for all parts of the body are given in *Progressive Exercise Therapy* (4th edition), by Colson and Collison, published by John Wright and Sons.

and then allows the heels to return to the floor again. The exercise is repeated after a brief pause.

Ex. 4. As the previous exercise, but the arms are not used to assist the movement; they hang by the sides or are placed in the 'hips-firm' position.

Ex. 5. As Ex. 3, but the player stands on one leg, with the foot of the other leg resting on a stool or chair behind him. (Fig. 12.) Several movements are carried out in succession, with brief rest periods between each movement; the other leg is then exercised.

Ex. 6. As previous exercise, but the arms are not used to assist the movement. *See* Ex. 4.

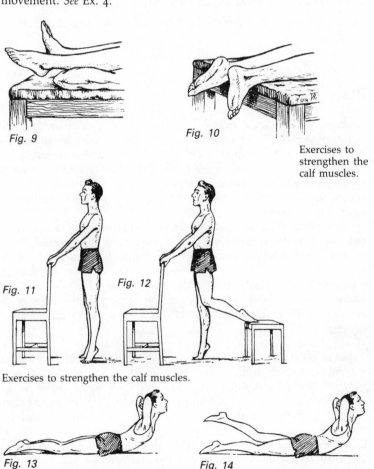

Fig. 9

Fig. 10

Exercises to strengthen the calf muscles.

Fig. 11

Fig. 12

Exercises to strengthen the calf muscles.

Fig. 13

Fig. 14

Exercises to strengthen the back muscles.

Progressive exercises for back muscles

Ex. 1. The player lies face downwards on the floor with his arms at his sides, palms facing upwards. He bends the trunk backwards as far as possible, at the same time turning the arms outwards strongly so that the palms face forwards. (Fig. 117, p. 178). He 'holds' the final position for a moment, and then allows the trunk and arms to return to their former position.

Ex. 2. As the previous exercise, but the hands are clasped behind the head. (Fig. 13).

Ex. 3. As Ex. 1, but the trunk movements are combined with a raising and lowering of each leg in turn. (Fig. 119, p. 178).

Ex. 4. As the previous exercise, but the hands are clasped behind the head. (Fig. 14).

Resisted exercises

Resisted exercises are extremely valuable in the intermediate and late stages of recovery after injury. They are able to bring about muscle hypertrophy in a way that is not possible with free movements. In addition, they are of considerable psychological value, for the incontrovertible evidence (as shown by regular testing) that the muscles are becoming progressively stronger is a great encouragement to the injured sportsman.

It is sometimes argued that resisted exercises are tedious and boring, but this depends on how the exercise programme is organized. If the patient is responsible for increasing the resistance whenever possible, keeping a careful check on the weights used and the number of repetitions, he is fully 'involved' in the best possible way, and his interest will be maintained. The periodic testing of the muscles to ascertain their maximum exercise efficiency also creates considerable interest.

Types of resistance. Resisted exercises consist of straightforward joint movements which are resisted by some form of apparatus, e.g. weights, weight-and-pulley circuits, and long spiral springs. In general, resistance by weights and weight-and-pulley circuits is better than spring resistance, because it can be measured more accurately.

Exercise technique. Resisted exercises should be performed smoothly and fairly slowly in such a way that the muscles work concentrically, statically and then eccentrically. Thus, in strengthening the quadriceps femoris muscle (Fig. 15a, p. 49), the patient extends the knee joint to

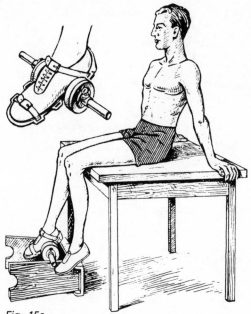

Fig. 15a

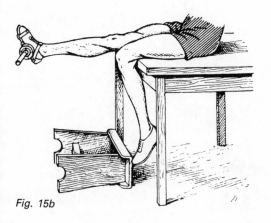

Fig. 15b

Weight-resisted exercise to strengthen the quadriceps muscle. Note the method of supporting the weight-shoe when the quadriceps is relaxed; this relieves the knee ligaments of strain.

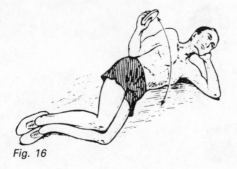

Fig. 16

Weight-resisted exercise to strengthen the outward rotator muscles of the shoulder joint.

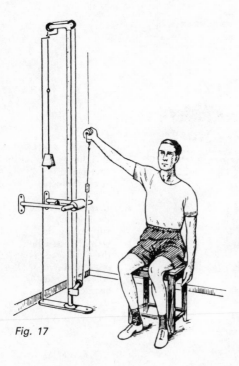

Fig. 17

The Armour Exerciser being used to strengthen the abductor muscles of the shoulder joint. The unit is no longer manufactured.

its full extent, 'holds' it in position for a moment, and then allows it to return to the starting position.

Relaxation. It is essential that some arrangement is made to ensure that the muscles can relax completely in the starting position and after each contraction. Fig. 15b, p. 49 shows how this can be done when a weight-boot is used.

If a weight-and-pulley unit is employed the circuit can be adjusted to achieve this effect in two ways: by the weight-bag resting on the floor at the beginning and end of the exercise, or by incorporating a simple relaxation stop into the circuit, so that it strikes a pulley sheave and takes the strain of the weight when the starting position is assumed.[2] *See* Fig. 17, p. 50.

Systems of training. Many different systems of resistance training are in use (p. 53). Some employ very heavy poundages and comparatively low repetitions. These are ideal for boosting the strength of normal muscles, but may prove harmful when used in the treatment of weak muscles and traumatized joints. On the other hand, it must be admitted that if the poundages are kept to a low figure, with repetitions at a comparatively high level, there will be little chance of bringing about muscle hypertrophy. This type of technique will promote the development of endurance rather than strength.

Strength technique. The resistance technique described here has been found extremely useful in practice over a long period of time.

Initial dosage. It has been found safe to exercise weak muscles against an *initial* resistance of 25 per cent of the greatest weight which they can lift ten times in succession at a normal controlled rate without marked discomfort or fatigue. The ten-times weight is known as the '10 Repetition Maximum' or '10 RM'; the smaller weight is known as the 'Minimum Exercise Weight'.

On the first day of treatment the muscles are exercised against the minimum exercise weight for a period of 4 minutes, a brief rest period being taken halfway through the exercise session. Thus the patient exercises continuously for 2 minutes, rests until his muscles feel capable of exercising again, and then exercises for another 2 minutes.

Progression. Progression in strength is brought about very gradually by increasing the minimum exercise weight by a quarter or half a pound when the patient finds that he has grown accustomed to the weight he has been lifting, and the effort no longer tires the muscles to any appreciable extent. (Some degree of fatigue is unavoidable if the resistance weight is of the poundage necessary to bring about

---

[2] Practical details of weight-and-pulley circuits are given in *Progressive Exercise Therapy* (4th edition), by Colson and Collison, published by John Wright and Sons.

muscle hypertrophy.) The weight increase is continued in this way until the resistance employed is found to be about 50 per cent of the 10 Repetition Maximum weight (which will also have increased, of course). The minimum exercise weight is then kept at this level until treatment is discontinued, the actual weight used being increased in direct proportion to the 10 RM. The 10 RM must be checked twice weekly to ascertain if it may be increased: an extremely important matter.

Progression in time is achieved by increasing the exercise time by one minute each day until the patient is exercising with the minimum exercise weight for 15 minutes before the rest pause, and 15 minutes after it. The length of the rest pause depends entirely on the degree of muscle fatigue.

On occasions it is helpful if two exercise periods are organized daily, provided that they are adequately spaced to avoid undue fatigue. A morning and afternoon session is ideal.

Advanced technique. When the muscles have reached a satisfactory state of redevelopment a more advanced exercise technique, combining both power and endurance training, can be used. This form of training has the advantage of preparing the muscles for normal function: short periods of activity against maximum stresses and prolonged periods of work against minimum stresses.

The technique is similar to that previously described, with the exception that two sets of lifts with the 10 RM are incorporated into the training schedule. Thus: (a) the 10 RM weight is lifted 10 times; (b) the minimum exercise weight (50 per cent of the 10 RM) is then lifted for the appropriate amount of time, complete with half-time rest pause; and (c) the 10 RM weight is lifted 10 times.

It is important to note that, although the patient may not be able to carry out the full number of repetitions during the second set of lifts with the 10 RM, he must be prepared to attempt as many lifts as possible. Unless this is done maximum hypertrophy of the muscle group being treated will not occur. Care must be taken that the over-enthusiastic patient does not attempt too much; this can easily lead to a joint effusion or muscle strain.

Exercise efficiency tests. It is important to check regularly the 10 RM weight of the corresponding sound muscle group, so that the relative weakness of the affected muscle group can be ascertained, and a standard set at which the patient can aim. The results should be plotted as a graph. In dealing with the trunk muscles, where this type of comparison is not possible, a known standard is determined by testing out normal subjects.

Each time the tests are made the same apparatus should be used. This is very important when weight-and-pulley circuits are employed:

the amount of frictional resistance offered by individual pulleys varies considerably, although if they are well constructed and lubricated frequently this should not be a big factor. The same applies, of course, when the circuits are used for exercises.

Testing. In assessing the 10 RM of a muscle group it is important for the patient to avoid trying out too many different poundages before arriving at the correct one. The muscles will become so fatigued by this preliminary work that it will be almost impossible to make an accurate test.

A useful way of determining the 10 RM is for the therapist to select a weight which he considers to be a reasonable resistance for the purpose of the test, and then ask the patient to make a *small* movement against its resistance. In this way the patient can try the effect of the weight on his muscles without using them sufficiently to produce fatigue. If he finds the weight is too much or too little (bearing in mind a series of 10 repetitions), the poundage is adjusted accordingly and the test is repeated.

When the patient considers that the correct weight has been found, he attempts the 10 full movements against it. No further tests are carried out if the therapist and patient are satisfied that the weight is adequate. If they are not satisfied the muscles are given a sufficient rest period before a further test is made.

Other methods of resistance training

Three main systems (based on the heavy resistance techniques used by bodybuilders and weight-lifters) are in use today: DeLorme and Watkins technique; Zinovieff or Oxford technique; and McQueen technique. These heavy resistance systems are mainly intended for use with weights, although they may be used equally well with weight-and-pulley circuits. Common to the three techniques is the 10 Repetition Maximum (10 RM), the maximum weight which can be lifted by the weak muscle group for ten repetitions only.

DeLorme and Watkins 'Fractional' Technique. The 10 RM resistance is increased gradually over three sets of repetitions. Thus:
Set 1: 10 lifts with half 10 RM
Set 2: 10 lifts with three-quarters 10 RM
Set 3: 10 lifts with 10 RM

Thirty lifts are performed daily, four times a week. Each week the 10 RM is progressed.

The system has the advantage of being simple to follow. Care is required in assessing the initial 10 RM, or the patient may be frustrated by finding it impossible to achieve the final full set of lifts.

Zinovieff or Oxford Technique. The 10 RM is *decreased* gradually over ten sets of repetitions. Thus:

Set 1: 10 lifts with 10 RM
Set 2: 10 lifts with 10 RM subtracting 1 lb.
Set 3: 10 lifts with 10 RM subtracting 2 lbs.
Set 4: 10 lifts with 10 RM subtracting 3 lbs.
Sets 5–10 continue in the same manner, weight being gradually subtracted from the 10 RM

A hundred lifts are carried out daily, five times a week. At each exercise session an attempt is made to progress the 10 RM.

Because of the high number of repetition sets, all with different weights, many patients and therapists find the system not only irritating but extremely time-consuming.

McQueen technique. The 10 RM resistance is *maintained*, without addition or subtraction, over four separate sets of lifts. Forty lifts are carried out three times a week. Progression is achieved by attempting to increase the 10 RM every one to two weeks.

In this system the overall workload is heavy, and the patient needs a great deal of determination to follow it conscientiously. Care is needed in assessing the initial 10 RM, or overloading of the muscles may result and the patient may not be able to complete the final set of lifts.

Alternative heavy resistance systems. Other heavy resistance systems have been developed by therapists and trainers with specialized knowledge of weight-training. The RM varies between 1 and 10, with 6 or 8 RM being common. The number of sets of lifts varies also. For maximum muscle development 6 repetitions, in six sets of lifts, is often advocated (36 lifts in all).

Many therapists with a background of weight-training consider that the generally accepted figure of 10 lifts per set could be replaced by a lower number, and suggest 6 as a suitable compromise. They consider that the patient's concentration and interest diminish over long sessions of muscle boosting.

Monitoring muscle strength. Two types of instrument have been developed for the accurate assessment of muscle strength: (1) a simple hand-held myometer, and (2) an isokinetic dynamometer.

The *hand-held myometer* has been developed by Penny and Giles Transducers of Christchurch, Dorset. Basically, the instrument is a device to measure the peak force applied by the therapist in resisting, and overcoming, the maximum contraction of a muscle group. The force is expressed in kilograms and the instrument has a recorded range of 0.1–30.00 kg, which may be seen on the digital readout display.

The myometer head, which incorporates a spreader applicator, utilizes the measuring element of a standard Penny and Giles transducer. The method of measuring consists of the deflection of a diaphragm in air. The deflection moves the wiper of a conductive plastic potentiometer.

To some degree the usefulness of the instrument is limited by the strength of the therapist in resisting the contractions of the patient's muscles. He needs to assume a very stable position when using the myometer, particularly when testing large powerful muscle groups, such as the quadriceps femoris and hamstrings.

The best-known *isokinetic dynamometer* is the Cybex II, now available in this country from Nomeq of Redditch. It can be used in sports medicine both in the redevelopment of specific muscle groups and in the promotion of endurance. It can also be employed to compare the function of the injured and uninjured limbs, and so provide accurate information on the patient's potential for recovery and improvement.

Since 1970 the isokinetic dynamometer has been used widely in North America and Sweden in the treatment and evaluation of injured athletes. In the UK, however, its use has been confined mainly to selective research projects, largely because of the high price of the equipment.

In essence the isokinetic dynamometer consists of a sophisticated electro-mechanical system comprising dynamometer, upper and lower body tables, and a chart recorder. This last prints out torque measured in foot-pounds and range of motion. A speed selector is also incorporated: it provides graduated resistance in both directions of the movement required.

The dynamometer itself is fully adjustable, and can be tilted or swivelled to accommodate itself to the axis of rotation of the movement which is being tested or exercised.

A recent addition to the isokinetic range of equipment is the fully computerized isokinetic dynamometer manufactured by the Chattecx Corporation of Chattanooga, Tennessee, USA.

Mobility exercises

Mobility exercises are used in association with strengthening exercises, although they may be started a little later. They consist of two main types: (1) Free movements of the joints, and (2) Auto-Assisted Active (Tension) exercises performed with cord-and-pulley circuits.

Free mobility exercises

At first the exercises consist of straightforward joint movements, e.g. bending and stretching of the ankle joints. As soon as possible they are progressed to movements which include a series of rhythmical presses. Rhythmical swinging movements are also used for the larger joints, such as the shoulder, hip and knee.

Exercise technique. The player is encouraged to move the stiff joint through as wide a range of movement as possible without producing too much pain. The movements should be performed smoothly and continuously. It is important that the movements should be confined as much as possible to the stiff joint, and that 'trick' movements should not be allowed to occur at the neighbouring sound joints.

Some examples of progressive mobility exercises[3] are given here.

Restoring ankle mobility

Ex. 1. From a half-lying position on a massage couch (Fig. 61, p. 114) the player alternately bends and stretches the stiff ankle joint as much as possible. The exercise is repeated 10 or 12 times; the joint is then rested for a few moments, and the exercise is repeated. It is helpful if the leg rests on a pillow, to keep the heel clear of the couch top.

The ankle of the sound leg may also be included in the exercise; this often helps to produce a better range of movement at the stiff joint. As one foot is bent up the other is pointed down, and *vice versa*. (Fig. 18.)

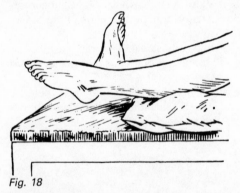

Fig. 18

Ex. 2. As the previous exercise, but movement is confined to the stiff joint. At the end of each upward and downward movement of the foot the player carries out a series of 3 or 4 rhythmical pressing movements. Thus he bends the foot up almost as far as it will go, lets it drop a little, pulls it up again (if possible, further than before), and repeats the process. It is important that the player is warned not to attempt to increase the range of movement if this causes a considerable amount of pain.

---

[3] *See* footnote 1, p. 46.

Ex. 3. The player rests the foot of the injured leg on a stool or chair top. He then makes a series of small-range pressing movements in a forward direction, as shown in Fig. 19a. The movements are usually performed for about 2 or 3 minutes with brief rest periods.

The exercise can also be carried out from the half-kneeling position, as shown in Fig. 19b.

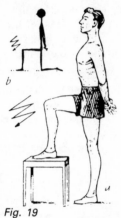

Fig. 19

Exercises to restore ankle mobility.

Increasing knee flexion

Ex. 1. From a half-lying position on a massage couch the player raises and lowers the thighs alternately, while the heels are kept in contact with the couch top. (Fig. 20). The exercise is performed for several minutes with short rest periods.

Ex. 2. The player sits on a wide bench or table with the thighs well supported and the feet clear of the ground. If the stiff knee will not flex to 90°, it should be flexed as much as possible and the foot supported on a stool, as shown in Fig. 21. The player stretches and bends the knees alternately in a rhythmical manner for several minutes.

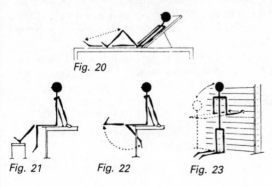

Fig. 20

Fig. 21   **Fig. 22**   **Fig. 23**

Exercises to restore knee mobility. Fig. 21 shows the starting position to use for alternate knee bending and stretching when the stiff knee will not flex to 90°.

Ex. 3. As the previous exercise, but the legs are swung vigorously forwards and backwards, knee flexion being well accentuated. (Fig. 22.) Ankle movements should reinforce the knee movements, plantar-flexion accompanying knee flexion and dorsiflexion accompanying knee extension, as indicated in Fig. 22.

Ex. 4. The player kneels in front of the wall-bars or a chair seat; he grasps a bar at hip level or rests his hands on the chair seat. He then attempts to sit back on his heels, using his arms to take some of the body-weight. (Fig. 23.) He takes the movement as far as possible, 'holds' the position for a moment, and then returns to the starting position. The exercise is repeated about 10 or 12 times.

Ex. 5. The player kneels on hands and knees (prone kneeling position) and moves the trunk backwards and forwards rhythmically, attempting to take the backward movements as far as the limited knee movement will allow. The exercise is repeated 10 or 12 times.

The exercise can be progressed by adding rhythmical pressing to a given count at the end of the backward movement.

Cord-and-pulley exercises

These exercises are usually reserved for stiff joints which have failed to respond to treatment by free mobility exercises. The stiff joint is linked to the corresponding sound joint by a simple cord-and-pulley circuit, the length of the cord being adjusted by means of the 'runners', so that it is reasonably taut and responsive to movement.

The patient moves the injured limb in the required direction, simultaneously moving the other limb in the appropriate direction so as to keep the circuit cord taut. *See* Figs. 24 and 25. When the injured joint enters the stiff painless zone of movement, and reaches the point where assistance is required, the patient endeavours to take the movement still further with the prime mover muscles: *at the same time* he reinforces them by exerting tension on the cord with the sound limb. On reaching the painful limit he 'holds' the position for a moment, and then returns the limbs to their starting position by a reversal of the previous movements. Throughout, the exercise should be performed smoothly and fairly slowly.

Fig. 24 shows the hamstrings being helped to flex a stiff knee joint with the assistance of the knee extensor muscles of the opposite side. Fig. 25 shows how assistance can be given to the elevator muscles of the right arm with the assistance of the depressor muscles of the left arm.

Cord-and-pulley exercises are usually performed for about 10 to 15 minutes at a time with short rest periods.

Avoiding passive movements. In using cord-and-pulley circuits it is

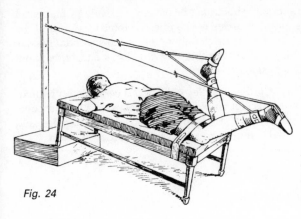

Arrangement of
cord-and-
pulley circuit to
restore knee
flexion.

Fig. 24

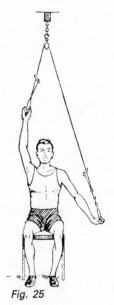

Cord-and-pulley circuit being
used to assist elevation of the
arm.

Fig. 25

important that a stiff joint should not be moved passively by the sound limb. The prime mover muscles of the affected joint *must* control the whole movement – the sound limb only reinforces their action. Passive movements to stiff joints irritate the joint structures and bring about the formation of adhesions.

Constructing circuits. Cord-and-pulley circuits can be made up without difficulty. The essentials consist of a pulley block with a 2 in. sheave, a swivel for the pulley hook, a length of sash cord, two handles, and two wooden or metal 'runners' to adjust the length of the cord.

Coordination exercises

After injury it is vital to restore the sportsman's confidence in his ability to move freely and safely when following his chosen sport. This is especially important when an athlete or player has been forced by injury to follow a very restricted physical routine or to abandon training altogether for several weeks. *See also* Training, p. 226.

Exercises which are valuable in this connection – particularly after injuries of the lower limb and trunk – in as much as they develop physical dexterity and neuromuscular coordination, are the rhythmical hopping and skipping exercises. Certain balance exercises which necessitate balance walking on raised apparatus, such as the rib of a balance bench or the broad side of a gymnasium beam, are also valuable in building up confidence. Increasing the height of the apparatus used, because of its psychological effect, disturbs the equilibrium of the subject.

Some specimen exercises for developing coordination are given here. Before they are used the patient should be thoroughly grounded in simple preparatory exercise techniques which pave the way for the more complex movements.

Preparatory activities

1. (a) Rhythmical hopping on alternate feet with or without the use of the arms, e.g. hopping with alternate toe placing forwards and sideways; (b) hopping with a rebound[4] on alternate feet, e.g. hopping with a rebound and opposite arm and knee raising forwards.

2. (a) Skipping, using both feet, either on the spot or 'travelling' –

---

[4] In hopping or skipping with rebound the subject springs up and down on his toes *twice*. The first spring consists of a strong plantar-flexion of the ankle(s); the landing is made on the toes and should be as light as possible. This is followed by another spring (the rebound jump), which is not quite so high as the first one.

moving forwards, backwards and sideways while skipping; (b) skipping with a rebound[4] jump, on the spot or 'travelling'; and (c) as previous exercise, with emphasis given to the height of the spring, e.g. high skip jump.

3. (a) Balance walking forwards and backwards along a straight line on the floor; (b) as previous exercise, but with opposite arm and knee raising forwards; and (c) balance walking forwards, backwards and sideways on rib of balance bench.

Progressive exercises

Hopping and skipping

1. Hopping with a rebound and alternate leg swinging in a circle. (Fig. 26.)

2. Hopping with a rebound and opposite arm and knee raising forwards.

3. Skipping: high skip jump with rebound – (a) on the spot (Fig. 27), and (b) 'travelling' forwards, backwards and sideways.

4. Skipping: (a) skip jump with rebound and alternate knee stretching forwards (Fig. 28), and (b) skip jump with rebound and alternate knee raising forwards (Fig. 29).

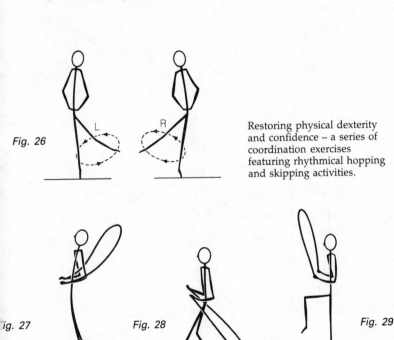

Fig. 26

Fig. 27

Fig. 28

Fig. 29

Restoring physical dexterity and confidence – a series of coordination exercises featuring rhythmical hopping and skipping activities.

Balancing

1. Balance walking forwards and backwards on rib of balance bench with opposite arm and knee raising forwards. (Fig. 30.) Progress to beam.

2. Balance walking forwards on rib of inclined balance bench. (Fig. 31.)

3. Standing on beam, with second beam arranged overhead – balance walking forwards and backwards, propelling a football on overhead beam. (Fig. 32.)

4. Standing on rib of balance bench – balance walking forwards, passing a ball from hand to hand. (Fig. 33.)

5. Standing on rib of balance bench – walking forwards, bouncing a football from side to side of bench. (Fig. 34.)

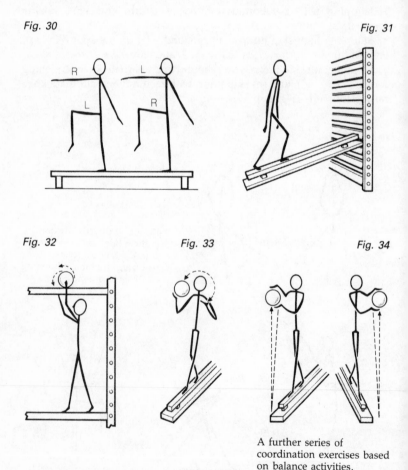

Fig. 30

Fig. 31

Fig. 32

Fig. 33

Fig. 34

A further series of coordination exercises based on balance activities.

Facilitation techniques

In recent years great interest has been shown by many therapists in the use of proprioceptive neuromuscular facilitation techniques (PNF) as a form of exercise therapy. The techniques, originally developed at the Kabat-Kaiser Institute in California, aim at obtaining maximum muscular activity by the employment of various forms of sensory stimuli and mass movement patterns.

PNF techniques were originally used for neurological conditions. Many therapists, however, now employ them in other fields, often substituting them for the more traditional forms of exercise therapy. While facilitation techniques may be used in the treatment of sports injuries as a re-educational process, their use cannot be considered essential or, indeed, necessary. The techniques are extremely time-consuming, and so far there is little evidence that the results claimed are not due largely to the intensity of treatment and the enthusiasm of the staff.

In brief, facilitation techniques involve putting muscles on the stretch (and so stimulating the stretch reflex), introducing traction and compression forces to the joints on which the muscles act, and administering pressure to the skin over the muscles in the line of the movement required. Maximum resistance is also applied to the muscles (which are encouraged to work in spiral and diagonal patterns, as in normal function), and great stress is laid on the patient's close participation in the techniques and in the effect of the therapist's voice as a verbal stimulus.

A full description of the practical application of PNF techniques is given in Hollis's *Practical Exercise Therapy* (2nd edition) Written by P. J. Waddington, an acknowledged expert in the field of neurophysiological movement, it includes detailed descriptions of patterns of movement for all parts of the body, together with clear illustrations of the various grasps to be used by the therapist in handling the patient.

A shorter, but extremely useful, account of PNF techniques is also included in Gardiner's *Principles of Exercise Therapy* (4th edition).

Part 2
Sports injuries and tests of fitness

Chapter 5
Injuries in sport

Archery

Archery is a relatively injury-free sport provided the normal safety precautions are followed. When too strong a bow is used the muscles of the shoulder-girdle are sometimes strained; the muscles most affected are the rhomboids and the upper and middle fibres of the trapezius. Fig. 53, p. 100. For treatment *see* p. 157.

Athletics

Sprinting, up to 400 yards

The most common injuries which occur in sprinting are: (1) Strains and tears of the hamstrings and calf muscles, (2) 'Pull' of the Achilles tendon, (3) Shin soreness, and (4) Bruising of the metatarsal heads.

Strains of hamstrings. Strains of the hamstrings can be as troublesome as tears, in that pain can be persistent and give rise when sprinting to muscle spasm; the spasm can lead to a severe tear. The runner is usually not aware of a mild strain until later in the day or the next morning. For treatment of strains, *see* p. 157.

Tears of hamstrings. Tears of the hamstrings usually occur in the middle of the muscle, or an inch or two below their origin on the ischial tuberosity. (Fig. 43, p. 89.) When a severe tear takes place the runner feels that he has been hit in the back of the thigh, and goes down like a 'shot bird'. Contrary to the average textbook description a gap is not felt at the site of the tear; rather, the bleeding from the tear forms a hard solid lump which is surrounded by local muscle spasm. If considerable bleeding has occurred 'bruising' or discoloration of the skin will appear behind the knee in a few days' time. The amount of bleeding does not necessarily indicate the severity of the injury; it is an indication of the size and number of blood vessels which have been torn.

In this injury, more than in any other muscle tear, the athlete carries a potentially weak spot for a very long time, probably months. The strain thrown upon the hamstrings by the sprinter is enormous, and not until the newly formed scar tissue has been thoroughly consolidated can he feel safe. *Treatment*: p. 158.

Strains and tears of the calf. Strains and tears of the calf muscles are not very common in sprinting; when they occur they clear up quickly and seldom give rise to trouble. *Treatment*: p. 165.

'Pulled' Achilles tendon. In sprinting a few fibres of the Achilles tendon are sometimes torn or 'pulled'; the pain, as in all tendon injuries, is out of all proportion to the severity of the injury. A small thickening, which is tender on pressure, is felt in the tendon about 1 to 2 in. above its insertion into the heel bone; creaking or crepitus may or may not be present.

In some cases the pain appears to be deep to the tendon, and although this may be because the injury is on the under aspect of the tendon, it is not unreasonable to suppose that the pain may be due to stretching of the binding connective tissue which holds the tendon in the most extraordinary bowed position when the athlete is on his toes. This belief is supported by the fact that considerable relief is given by applying a few turns of elastoplast round the lower part of the leg at the level of the injury; the relief of pain is greater than that obtained in cases where there is clear evidence of torn fibres.

Rupture of Achilles tendon. Complete rupture of the Achilles tendon is rare; when it occurs it is frequently unassociated with violent exercise, and seems to be due to lack of muscular coordination, e.g. an athlete was trotting between two hurdles when the tendon ruptured completely. *Treatment*: p. 168.

Shin soreness or 'shin splints'. This condition can occur in all runners, but is commoner in sprinters. There is acute pain on pressure along the lower two-thirds of the inner border of the tibia. (Fig. 37, p. 84.) Walking and training are painful, and in extreme cases the leg is painful when at rest; usually the pain is not felt during the actual race, especially in the shorter distances. In a few isolated (and acutely painful) cases shin soreness has been known to persist during the race.

Doubtless the cause of shin soreness is the continual pounding on a hard track or surface. It is not connected with muscle attachments, because there are no attachments on the lower third of the tibia where the pain is greatest. Cross-country runners whose pace is slower and who spend much of their running time on grass or ploughed land are much less likely to suffer from shin soreness. Some athletes seem to be particularly susceptible and predisposed to it, and they get frequent recurrences despite careful and progressive training. The pathology does not seem to be understood, but the condition strongly resembles a traumatic periostitis.

Treatment. No treatment appears to be of much value. The Americans have tried supporting the ankle in plantar-flexion with strips of strapping which pass under the heel and up the sides of the leg; the strips are held in position by bands of strapping which are applied transversely round the leg. Such a support acts as a shock-absorber or foot sling, but does not seem to be particularly efficacious.

Oddly enough, frictional massage over the affected area often gives relief, probably by relieving congestion. It is difficult to believe that massage can have a curative effect on shin soreness, however; if the condition is a periostitis, as suspected, one would expect massage to aggravate it.

Training. The athlete should be advised to cut his training to a minimum, to run on grass and avoid training on hard surfaces.

Bruising of metatarsal heads. The bruising may or may not accompany a dropping of the transverse arch of the foot (p. 108), frequently not. When running a felt or sponge-rubber pad should be worn; a considerable thickness of protective padding, up to ⅝ in., is necessary to give relief in some cases. The condition will clear up without further treatment in about two or three weeks.

Long-distance running

Long-distance runners come up against a variety of conditions which can only be described as over-use irritations and inflammations; it is noticeable that these have increased very much since the war, especially among runners who do much of their training on hard roads. The increase is no doubt due to the change in the mode of training during recent years. Until the war many runners trained only three times a week and were always on their guard to avoid becoming stale. The change of attitude is probably due to the success of such runners as Zatopek and Pirie who exploded the bogey of staleness by putting in a tremendous amount of training, and running as much as 100 miles a week. It has now become common for athletes, especially middle-distance and long-distance runners, to do likewise, and there has been a marked improvement in performance.

The commonest over-use conditions in middle- and long-distance runners are: (1) Painful feet and knees, (2) Tendinitis and teno-synovitis, (3) Bursitis, and (4) Fatigue or stress fracture.

Painful feet. No specific condition can be found. Tenderness or pain on pressure may or may not be present; when present it is not particularly acute. The same applies to passive movements of the joints of the feet.

Painful knees. Again no specific condition can be discovered. Passive and non-weight-bearing movements of the knees are complete and painless. Sometimes an area of tenderness is found on the outer side of the knee, some 3 in. above the joint line. Other points of pain are the inner and outer margins of the patella.

Tendinitis and teno-synovitis. Tendons and muscles are seldom torn in long-distance running, but a true over-use tendinitis of the Achilles tendon or the peroneal tendons (Fig. 38, p. 84) occurs. In the case of the Achilles tendon there is a marked 'wash-leather' creaking or crepitus, tenderness and congestion. Tendinitis may also develop in the hamstring tendons behind the knee. For treatment of tendinitis and teno-synovitis *see* p. 157.

Fatigue or stress fracture. The commonest site of fatigue or stress fracture in the athlete is the lower end of the fibula, about 1½ to 2 in. above the malleolus. (Fig. 35, p. 83.) In the early stages an X-ray will seldom reveal the presence of the fracture. It has been suggested that owing to the stress and strain thrown upon the bone repair occurs before the bone actually fractures.

Because of the absence of injury fatigue fractures of the fibula are often regarded as strains of the peronei muscles; threatened fatigue of the tibia is frequently mistaken for shin soreness. It must always be remembered that shin soreness disappears during the actual race, but in fatigue fracture the pain becomes worse and worse as the event proceeds – sometimes it becomes unbearable and the athlete has to drop out of the race. Strapping seldom helps; in fact it often seems to make the condition worse.

Rest from active exercise is the only treatment, once conclusive evidence of a stress fracture has been obtained; the period of inactivity may last for as long as 5 months.

'March' fracture. See p. 209.

Hurdling

'Pulled' hamstrings are fairly common. Strains and tears of the following muscles also occur in hurdling: rectus femoris and the hip flexors of the leading leg (Fig. 42, p. 88), and the adductor longus muscle of the trailing leg. See Fig. 44, p. 90.

'Clicking' hip. A few hurdlers develop a 'clicking' hip which seems to result from performing hurdling exercises with undue vigour. A click can be felt and heard during active circumduction (circling) of the hip when the thigh is passing from the abducted or sideways position to the midline of the body. The click may be due to slipping of a tendinous expansion over the bony prominence of the greater trochanter of the femur.

'Clicking' hip is not painful and does not handicap the athlete; he must be assured that the condition does not signify any underlying injury or disease.

High jumping

Bruising of the metatarsal heads is a frequent injury. Treatment consists of applying a felt or sponge-rubber pad behind the heads (*see* p. 109).

Long jumping

Long jumpers tend to get bruised heels from coming down hard on the take-off board. For treatment *see* p. 111. They also suffer from sprinting injuries (p. 67).

Discus-throwing

Rotation strains of the back sometimes occur. For treatment *see* p. 179.

Javelin-throwing

The main injuries consist of 'tennis elbow' and rotation strains of the back. For treatment *see* pp. 195 and 179.

Weight-putting

This is about the most trouble-free event in athletics. Minor strains of the shoulder-girdle and back muscles occasionally occur, and it has been known for a weight-putter to fracture a metatarsal bone from sheer muscular exertion. For treatment of strains *see* pp. 179 and 205.

Badminton

The injuries are similar to those of tennis. *See* p. 78.

Baseball

The hamstrings are sometimes strained or torn when sprinting for 'home plate'. Sprains of the ankle are common when 'sliding into base', especially when the forward velocity of the player is high and his foot position is dangerous. 'Sliding into base' also produces bruised heels and metatarsal heads, and sprains of the fingers and wrist: the hand is forced back on impact when checking the slide into base.

Pitchers often develop 'tennis elbow' and strains of the lumbar muscles. Most long-ball hitters sustain injuries from time to time; the most common injuries are 'tennis elbow' (due to too much explosive hitting without correct 'follow through'), sprains of the knee and wrist, and strains of the lumbar muscles. Wrist sprains are the bugbear of lazy 'wrist hitters' who try to deal with fast, inswinging balls; the hand is jarred backwards at the wrist.

Treatment. Strains and tears of hamstrings, pp. 157 and 158; sprained ankle, p. 113, knee, p. 133, fingers and wrist, pp. 186, 189; bruised heel and metatarsal heads, pp. 111 and 108; 'tennis elbow', p. 195; and lumbar back strains, p. 179.

Basketball

Sprains of the ankle are common in basketball because of the amount of running involved and the constant changes of direction. The knee is also sprained, but less frequently. Handling the ball often gives rise to sprains of the fingers.

Treatment. Sprained ankle, p. 113, knee, p. 133, and fingers, p. 186.

Bodybuilding

See p. 79.

Boxing

Injuries of the face, scalp and ear are common in boxing and include lacerations and bruises (e.g. 'cauliflower ear' and 'black eye') and fracture of the nose. Other injuries consists of bruising of the trunk, shoulder and arm muscles, sprains of the ankle and knee, and fractures of the metacarpal bones of the hand: the metacarpal bone of the thumb is particularly likely to be injured. Concussion may also occur as a result of a head injury (p. 219).

Because distance running is an essential part of the boxer's training he is also subject to the injuries of the long-distance runner (p. 69).

Treatment. Anodal galvanism (p. 39) is of great value in the early treatment of 'cauliflower ear' and 'black eye'; it reduces the swelling and disperses the bruising. For treatment of muscle bruising *see* p. 167. The treatment of sprains of the ankle and knee is dealt with on pp. 113 and 133, and the principles of fracture treatment are discussed on p. 209.

Cricket

A number of cricket injuries can rightly be described as 'occupational injuries', and are particularly troublesome because the player has to return to the game and perform the very movements which produced the injuries. The fast bowler is particularly likely to suffer in this respect, and may develop strains and tears of the rectus femoris muscle, the hip flexors or adductors, according to his style of bowling. For treatment *see* pp. 157 and 163. Bruised heels are also common (p. 111).

'Thrower's shoulder'. This is one of the most troublesome injuries of cricketers. It is usually very difficult to pin-point the damaged structures, but it is possible that the supraspinatus or biceps tendon is involved; the sub-deltoid bursa may also be injured. Frequently the player can bowl but is unable to throw hard; this applies particularly to an overarm throw. Slow movements of the shoulder may be painless, but the violent and 'explosive' action of throwing produces a most acute and almost paralysing pain. During the winter the condition appears to clear up completely, but at the first throw of the next season it is quite possible that the symptoms will recur. Treatment should be based on that suggested for tears of the supraspinatus muscle and sub-deltoid bursitis. *See* pp. 205 and 204.

Fencing

Fencing is a relatively injury-free sport provided the normal safety precautions are observed. Occasionally the quadriceps or calf muscle groups of the forward leg are strained. For treatment *see* p. 157. Sometimes, too, the medial ligament of the rear knee is sprained (p. 133).

Fives

Fives gives rise to two injuries which are not found in any other sport:

(1) Bruised palm, and (2) 'Seizing up' of the arm and forearm muscles. .

Bruised palm. Protection from bruising is the only answer to this problem. Players usually have their own pet forms of protection; these include padding the inside of the glove with felt, sponge-rubber, a slice of beef or even plasticine.

'Seizing up' of arm and forearm muscles. The condition affects the arm, especially the triceps region, and the upper part of the forearm. The player complains of excessive stiffness, which is similar to that experienced by a runner at the start of training. The stiffness occurs, however, as the result of excessive training; the muscles feel hard and turgid; they are painful during play and slow down the movements of the arm. The condition is probably a mild muscle inflammation or myositis.

Treatment. The stiffness improves when the player cuts down on training and play. General massage of the arm and forearm is often helpful.

Football

Rugby. Practically any injury can occur in rugby football and the upper limb and trunk are involved as much as the lower limb. Common injuries include: sprains of ligaments; strains, tears and bruising of muscles; dislocation of the shoulder joint and subluxation of the acromio-clavicular joint; tears of the semilunar cartilages of the knee; fractures of the leg, ribs, wrist and hand; and concussion.

Treatment. Sprains, *see* individual injuries, pp. 112 to 185; muscle and tendon injuries, pp. 156, 179 and 204; injuries of the semilunar cartilages, p. 152; dislocation of the shoulder, p. 201; acromio-clavicular subluxation, p. 198; fractures, p. 209; and concussion, p. 219.

Soccer. Soccer injuries are mainly confined to the lower limb, and consist of: sprains of the ankle and knee; strains, tears and bruising of muscles and tendons (particularly of the rectus femoris muscle and the Achilles tendon); and tears of the semilunar cartilages of the knee. Concussion sometimes occurs. For treatment of injuries *see* above.

Golf

There are three common golfing injuries: (1) 'Golfer's elbow', (2) Sprain of the medial ligament of the knee, and (3) Rotational strains of the back muscles. 'Golfer's elbow' (p. 195) is an over-use condition which is brought about by the combined movement of gripping and the swing-through action of the arm. The knee sprain is caused by a sudden rotational stress when 'driving' the ball; the back muscles are strained in the same way.

Treatment. 'Golfer's elbow', p. 196; knee sprain, p. 133; and back strains, p. 179.

Hockey

All the usual injuries can occur in hockey, including blows on the knee and shin.

Blows on the knee. If the player receives a really hard blow on the knee with the ball or stick he may develop a severe haemarthrosis (bleeding into the joint); if the knee is not aspirated the reabsorption of the fluid is a long and tedious business. *See* also p. 149.

Blows on the shin. Normally blows on the shin do not cause much trouble, except for the acute pain on pressure; this can always be dealt with adequately by protective padding. A shin injury should always be kept under observation, however, because it may develop into an infective periostitis, even though there is no apparent break in the skin. After a few days the affected part gets more painful on pressure, swelling or oedema develops over and around the site of injury, and there may be evidence of infected lymphatic vessels. The player may feel unwell and have a slightly elevated temperature. Infected periostitis nearly always occurs in the lower third of the tibia, where the bone is subcutaneous.

Most of the shin blows which occur in hockey result in the formation of a bruise under the periosteum (subperiosteal haematoma), and usually leave behind a nodule of bone at the site of the bleeding.

Judo and 'applied' judo

Judo. Judo injuries occur mainly because of incorrectly controlled falls. The most common injuries consist of bruising of the shoulder and trunk muscles and synovitis of the knee.

'Applied' judo. 'Applied' judo is widely used in the police and prison services and by the Armed Forces. It gives rise to a greater number of injuries than judo, especially when it is first taken up. The upper limb is chiefly involved, because of the nature of the various 'locks', 'holds' and 'throws'. Strains and sprains of the shoulder, elbow and wrist are common; dislocation of the shoulder sometimes occurs. Incorrectly controlled falls cause muscle bruising and synovitis of the knee, as in judo.

Treatment. Muscle bruising, p. 157; synovitis of knee, p. 148; strains and sprains, pp. 112 to 185; dislocation of the shoulder, p. 201.

Riding

Rider's strain. Riding always throws great strain on the adductor muscles of the thigh. When this strain is accentuated, as for example when a horse refuses a jump, the adductor longus (Fig. 44, p. 90) is strained or torn; if the horse refuses to the left the left adductor longus is injured, and *vice versa*. For treatment *see* p. 164.

Falls. Almost any injury can occur as a result of a fall; the most common conditions consist of bruising and tearing of the trunk muscles and fractures of the clavicle and skull. Severe head injuries (e.g. fractures with haemorrhage within the skull) are fortunately rare; they occur, for instance, when a horse kicks its rider in a fall.

Rowing

Apart from septic fingers and boils on the buttocks, the common injuries are: (1) Teno-synovitis of the extensor tendons of the wrist, (2) Strains of the back muscles, and (3) 'Nipping' strains of the lumbar discs.

Teno-synovitis of wrist extensor tendons (p. 94). The condition is probably caused by the oarsman gripping the oar too tightly and not allowing the wrist to relax sufficiently. One would expect the condition to be commoner in inexperienced oarsmen, but this is not so.

Treatment. Opinion on treatment is divided. Some doctors recommend heat and massage; others prefer to immobilize the wrist in a plaster cast. A third group suggest immobilizing the wrist in a removable plaster cast so that heat, gentle massage and movement can be given once or twice daily; this compromise often gives excellent results.

Strains of back muscles. The back muscles are strained either in the lumbar region or higher up the spine, just below the inferior angle of the scapula. For treatment *see* p. 179.

'Nipping' strains of lumbar discs. A number of back injuries are very suggestive of disc injuries (p. 172). The constant forward movement of the spine may well act as a compression stress. For treatment *see* p. 174.

Sculling

Any of the injuries of rowing can occur in sculling, but are less frequent. A common condition which occurs in sculling (but is seldom seen in rowing) consists of a severe swelling of the forearm. The individual complains that his forearm 'blows up' while he is sculling, and that sometimes the swelling is so severe that he is unable to continue in the race. When he is seen an hour or so after he has left the river the forearm muscles are slightly swollen, hard and turgid.

The condition is probably the outcome of excessive active and static muscle work, with insufficient relaxation. Having one scull per hand renders it more difficult (as compared with rowing) to relax the forearm muscles, and it would seem that far more control of the scull is necessary in the recovery of the stroke than in rowing.

Treatment. No specific form of physiotherapy seems to be of much value in this condition, although massage of the forearm muscles is helpful in dispersing the residual stiffness.

Ski-ing

Ski-ing injuries are mainly confined to the knee, leg and ankle. The most common causes consist of the skis 'sticking', crossing or deviating (and the body continuing to move), so that the lower limb is subjected to a violent rotational strain.

The medial ligament of the knee is frequently sprained severely or completely ruptured; the cruciate ligaments of the knee are also sometimes torn. Severe sprains of the ankle ligaments are common, and are often associated with fractures of the fibula. Fractures of the tibia and fibula are also common.

Treatment. Knee injuries, pp. 133 and 145; sprained ankle, p. 113; principles of fracture treatment, p. 209.

Squash rackets

This is a surprisingly accident-free sport, considering the speed of the game and the agility required. Occasionally the heels and metatarsal heads are bruised; sometimes, too, sprains of the fingers occur when the player crashes into the wall of the court.

Squash is a useful rehabilitation activity for many of the lower-limb injuries which occur in the more violent games.

Treatment. Bruising of heels and metatarsal heads, pp. 111 and 109; finger sprains p. 186.

Swimming and diving

Swimming. Strains and sprains of muscles and joints are rare in swimming because of the supporting medium of the water and the fact that the body is not fixed during movement. Arm injuries (chiefly bruising) can occur in racing, however, due to violent contact with the bath-end when finishing or making a turn; this happens frequently in back crawl racing. For treatment of bruising *see* p. 157 and 167.

Diving. In all forms of diving from a spring-board the inexperienced diver may make contact with the vibrating board on his descent into the water. This is a common occurrence, and usually results only in grazing of the skin and superficial bruising.

High diving can give rise to very severe injuries. Internal abdominal injuries have been known to occur from incorrect entry ('belly-flop'). An inexperienced diver diving into an insufficient depth of water may sustain head, neck or facial injuries through striking the bottom of the bath. This may cause concussion, fractured skull or fracture-dislocation of the neck (resulting in paralysis of all four limbs). It is worth noting that fracture-dislocation of the neck occurs when the forehead is struck against the bottom and the neck is bent backwards (extension).

Tennis

The main 'occupational injuries' consist of: (1) 'Tennis elbow' (p. 194), (2) Bruised heels and metatarsal heads (pp. 111 and 108), and (3) Strains and tears of the calf and abdominal muscles (pp. 156 and 179).

When the abdominals are injured the 'straight' muscles may be affected, but the oblique muscles of the right side are far more likely to be injured if the player serves with his right arm. It is difficult to know whether the muscles are injured when the player stretches backwards to make the service, or during the stroke when the abdominals contract strongly.

Weight-lifting, weight-training and bodybuilding

Weight-lifting and weight-training. It is important to differentiate between competitive weight-lifting (where competitors are endeavouring to lift maximum poundages on certain selective lifts) and weight-training, which offers a much wider range of lifting exercises or movements against resistance. Competitive weight-lifting is naturally more hazardous than weight-training, because of the maximum effort made to elevate very heavy poundages.

The most common injuries which occur in both weight-lifting and weight-training are: strain of the forearm extensor muscles at the elbow ('tennis elbow'), and strains of the lumbar back muscles. Knee sprains sometimes occur.

'Tennis elbow' (p. 194) is brought about by practising certain types of triceps stretch exercises over a long period of time, and using too heavy a weight. The exercises which are particularly likely to give rise to trouble are the *Single arm seated triceps stretch with dumbell* and the *Bent-arm pullover on bench*. These exercises are widely practised by weight-trainers; when they are used it is important that they should be practised for a week or two only. For treatment of 'tennis elbow' *see* p. 195.

Lumbar back strains occur because the back is not kept straight during a lift, but is allowed to bend slightly. This happens often in the Press and the Squat. For treatment of back strains *see* p. 179.

Knee sprains may result from practising the Snatch. The exercise is widely recommended as a coordination exercise for all forms of sport, although it is difficult to understand why. It is an extremely difficult exercise to perform correctly, and one which can only be learned by individual tuition.

Bodybuilding. Good results, free from injury, are achieved by practising wide-range joint movements with adequate poundages. Naturally considerable physical effort and concentration are required.

Some bodybuilders attempt to get quicker results by practising half- or even quarter-range movements with excessively heavy weights. Inevitably this leads to sprains of ligaments and muscle strains. Many top-line bodybuilders have discovered this and quickly abandoned this form of training.

Inguinal hernia or rupture

Inguinal hernia or rupture is a real bogey to many sportsmen, particularly to bodybuilders, weight-trainers and -lifters. At first the hernia consists of a small lump or swelling in the groin; later it increases in size and may spread into the scrotum. The swelling often disappears when the individual lies down, but reappears when he stands upright, especially when he coughs.

The hernia consists of a small amount of gut or fat from the abdomen. It is pushed through a natural canal-like deficiency in the lower edge of the abdominal muscles by a sudden rise of pressure in the abdomen, such as occurs in coughing or any movement in which the abdominals are used strongly.

A hernia or rupture can happen to anyone, whatever his degree of physical fitness. It is more likely to occur in men whose abdominals are weak, who are employed in heavy industry, and who do not observe the correct technique of lifting.

Preventing a rupture. To safeguard himself against the occurrence of an inguinal hernia the sportsman must build up strong abdominal muscles, and pay particular attention to the obliques. In addition he must try to avoid movements which throw a *sudden* severe strain on the abdominals. Lastly, it is essential that he keeps his back straight when lifting heavy weights.

Treatment. When an inguinal hernia has occurred the doctor may advise an operation or the wearing of a truss. For young and middle-aged men who are physically fit an operation is most often chosen; the truss is usually reserved for those who are not fit enough to undergo an operation.

Chapter 6
Testing for injury and fitness

When the soft structures of the body are injured the therapist or the trainer must be able to test their normal function. He is then in a position (a) to determine whether the joints or the muscles have been injured, (b) to localize treatment accurately, and (c) to decide whether the player is fit enough to resume training when the injury appears to have recovered.

Functional tests for the main joints and muscles are described in this chapter, together with an outline of the basic anatomy of the structures involved.

Functional tests

Assessing the injury. In general local pain produced by a passive movement[1] indicates a ligamentous or joint injury; local pain produced by a resisted movement indicates a muscular injury.

Testing a joint. Each ligament is tested by the therapist moving the joint passively in such a way that the ligament is put on the stretch.

Testing muscles. The individual muscle groups are tested by the player using them against the therapist's resistance.

When the more superficial structures are involved the site of the injury is located by careful palpation.

Testing for fitness. The same passive and active tests are carried out. *See p. 227.*

1: Testing the ankle and its muscles

Basic anatomy

The ankle joint consists of the lower ends of the tibia and fibula, which

---

[1] Passive movements are those performed on the player by the therapist while the player's muscles are completely relaxed.

form a deep mortice, and the talus bone of the foot, as shown in Fig. 35. The talus is held in the mortice by a capsular ligament, which is reinforced by two strong ligaments: (*a*) the lateral ligament, which lies on the outer side of the joint and has three bands of fibres (Fig. 60, p. 112), and (*b*) the medial ligament, which lies on the inner side and also has three bands of fibres (Fig. 36). The capsule is lined by a synovial membrane.

Ankle movements. Two movements only occur at the ankle: dorsiflexion (an upward movement of the foot) and plantar-flexion (a downward movement of the foot). *See* Fig. 18, p. 56. Dorsiflexion is brought about mainly by the tibialis anterior and the toe extensors. (Fig. 37.) Plantar-flexion is performed by the calf, the tibialis posterior and the peronei. (Fig. 38).

Foot movements. In the foot the medial and lateral ligaments of the ankle are attached to some of the main bones, as shown in Fig. 36 and Fig. 60, p. 112. These bones form the joints which allow the foot to turn inwards (inversion) and outwards (eversion). Inversion is produced mainly by the tibialis anterior and posterior, and eversion by the peronei.

Testing the ankle and foot

Lateral ligament (Fig. 60, p. 112). The player is in half-lying (Fig. 61, p. 114). The therapist grasps the foot firmly with one hand; with the other he holds the leg just above the ankle.

Front band. The therapist passively plantar-flexes the ankle, and then turns the foot into inversion. If pain is experienced the front band should be palpated until the site of the injury is found.

Middle band. As above, but the foot is first *slightly* plantar-flexed and then inverted.

Back band. The therapist passively dorsiflexes the ankle, and then inverts the foot. If pain is felt the band must be palpated for the area of injury.

Medial ligament (Fig. 36). The ligament is tested in a similar manner to the lateral ligament, with the exception that eversion is substituted for inversion. For example, to test the front band the therapist passively plantar-flexes the ankle and then everts the foot.

Testing the leg muscles

For these tests the player is in half-lying (Fig. 61, p. 114).

Plantar-flexor muscles (Fig. 38). The player plantar-flexes the ankle against the resistance of the therapist's hand, which is placed against the sole of the foot; the therapist's other hand holds the leg a little above the ankle.

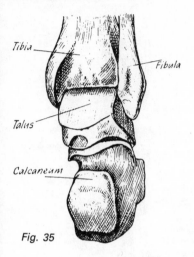

Tibia
Fibula
Talus
Calcaneum

Fig. 35

Back view of the right ankle joint showing the deep mortice formed by the lower ends of the tibia and fibula.

If pain is produced by the movement the muscles at the back of the leg should be palpated for the site of the injury. Fairly common sites are: (*a*) attachment of calf muscles to femur, (*b*) belly of calf, (*c*) insertion of calf into the Achilles tendon, and (*d*) the Achilles tendon.

Dorsiflexor muscles (Fig. 37). As previous test, but the ankle is dorsi-flexed against the therapist's resistance; the hand rests on top of the foot. A common site of injury is the junction of the tibialis anterior muscle with its tendon.

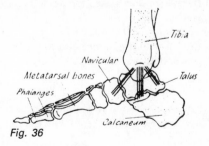

Tibia
Navicular
Metatarsal bones
Talus
Phalanges
Calcaneum

Fig. 36

Diagram of the medial ligament of the right ankle joint.

Tendinitis. Pain on dorsiflexion of the ankle is sometimes caused by an inflammation of the tendons of the long extensor muscles of the toes (Fig. 37). The specific test for this condition consists of first resisting extension of the four outer toes, and then of the great toe.

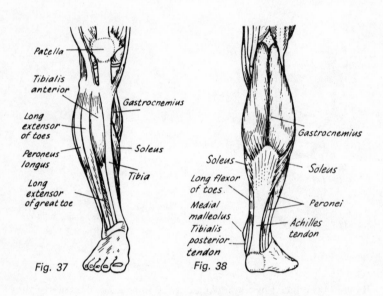

Fig. 37

Fig. 38

Front view of the muscles of the right leg.

Back view of the right leg showing the muscles of the calf: gastrocnemius and soleus. The tibialis posterior muscle lies deep to the calf; the tendon only is shown here.

Invertor muscles. To test the tibialis posterior (which is covered by the calf muscles) the player plantar-flexes the ankle; he then inverts the foot against the therapist's resistance. Tibialis anterior (Fig. 37), is tested in a similar manner, but the player dorsiflexes the ankle before inverting the foot.

In giving resistance the therapist grasps the forepart of the foot firmly with one hand; he holds the leg with the other hand to prevent it from twisting and taking part in the foot movements.

Evertor muscles. The peronei (Fig. 38) are tested in a similar manner to the tibialis posterior, with the exception that the foot is everted instead of being inverted.

2: Testing the knee and its muscles

Basic anatomy

The knee joint is formed by the junction of the lower end of the femur, the upper end of the tibia, and the patella. (Fig. 39.) The femur and tibia are bound together by a capsular ligament and two strong bands, the cruciate ligaments, which lie deep inside the joint and cross each other. (Fig. 40.) The patella is held in position on the front of the thigh by the quadriceps muscle, as shown in Fig. 42, p. 88.

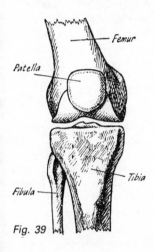

Fig. 39   Bones forming the right knee joint.

Ligaments. The capsule is reinforced by the medial ligament, which lies on the inner side of the knee, and the lateral ligament, which is situated on the outer side. (Fig. 41.) The medial ligament has both deep and superficial sets of fibres; the deep fibres are attached to the medial semilunar cartilage. *See* Fig. 91, p. 132.

Semilunar cartilages. The upper end of the tibia is covered by two crescent-shaped pieces of fibro-cartilage, the menisci or semilunar cartilages, which are attached to the bone by their outer borders and horn-like ends. (Fig. 40.) The functions of the semilunar cartilages are described on p. 151.

Synovial membrane. This lines the capsule and forms a large pouch which lies under the tendon of the quadriceps muscle (Fig. 41); it extends for about three finger-breadths above the upper border of the patella. Fringes of synovial membrane project into the joint.

Synovial sacs or bursae. Small sacs of synovial fluid are found at different points around the knee joint, particularly at areas where the tendons pass close to bones; they act as cushions. An important sac lies under the tendon of the semimembranosus muscle at the back of the knee. After a synovial effusion of the knee (p. 148) this sac often remains tense and swollen, because it communicates directly with the joint.

Knee movements. These consists of (a) hinge-like movements of flexion and extension, and (b) twisting movements, which can only take place when the joint is bent. During the twisting movements the unattached parts of the semilunar cartilages move to a certain extent on top of the tibia. Any excess of cartilage movement when the knee is bearing weight may tear the cartilage and cause 'locking' of the joint. *See* p. 151.

Flexion is brought about by the hamstrings, extension by the quadriceps, and inward rotation mainly by the hamstrings and popliteus. Outward rotation is performed by the biceps femoris.

Testing the joint

Medial ligament (Fig. 41, p. 87). With the player in half-lying (Fig. 61, p. 114) the therapist grasps the leg above the ankle and places the other hand on the outside of the knee. He then attempts to press the joint into the 'knock-knee' position by drawing the leg outwards and pressing the thigh inwards. *During this movement the knee should be kept in slight flexion.* If pain is felt during the test the medial ligament must be palpated carefully to find the site of the injury. It is important to remember that the medial ligament limits outward rotation of the knee, and this should be tested with the joint in no more than 90°.

Lateral ligament (Fig. 41). The test is a reversal of the previous one. The hand which rests on the knee is placed on the inside of the joint, and the knee is pressed into the 'bow-leg' position.

Cruciate ligaments (Fig. 40, p. 87). The knee is bent to about 40°, with the player is half-lying (Fig. 61, p. 114); the muscles acting on the joint must be completely relaxed. The therapist sits on the foot of the bent leg, and grasps the upper end of the tibia with both hands. The tibia is pressed backwards; any pain produced by this movement indicates an injury of the posterior cruciate ligament. The tibia is then pulled forwards; pain indicates an injury of the anterior cruciate ligament. It should be noted that the cruciate ligaments limit inward rotation of the joint, and should be tested with the knee flexed to about 40°.

An increased range of forward-backward movement of the knee (in comparison with the sound joint) results from a severe sprain or complete tear of one or both cruciate ligaments, and is permanent. For treatment *see* p. 146.

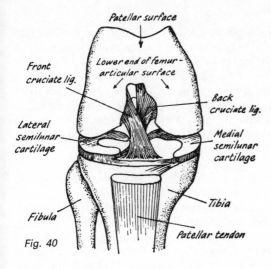

Front cruciate lig.

Patellar surface

Lower end of femur - articular surface

Back cruciate lig.

Lateral semilunar cartilage

Medial semilunar cartilage

Tibia

Fibula

Patellar tendon

Fig. 40

Diagrammatic impression of the interior of the right knee joint from the front to show the cruciate ligaments and the semilunar cartilages.

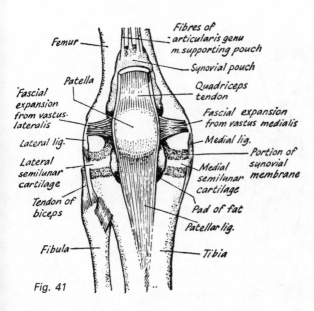

Femur

Fibres of articularis genu m. supporting pouch

Patella

Synovial pouch

Fascial expansion from vastus. lateralis

Quadriceps tendon

Fascial expansion from vastus medialis

Lateral lig.

Medial lig.

Lateral semilunar cartilage

Portion of synovial membrane

Medial semilunar cartilage

Tendon of biceps

Pad of fat

Patellar lig.

Fibula

Tibia

Fig. 41

Front view of the right knee joint to show the position of the synovial pouch.

Testing the thigh muscles

Quadriceps (Fig. 42). The player takes up the half-lying position (Fig. 61, p. 114) with the knee joint flexed to a right angle. The therapist places one hand on the leg, just above the ankle, and asks the player to extend the knee. Pain occurring during the movement indicates an injury of the quadriceps group of muscles. The site of the injury must be found by palpating the muscles. If the injury is thought to be localized to the rectus femoris (Fig. 42) the player should be asked to perform a *combined* movement of knee extension and hip flexion against the therapist's resistance.

Hamstrings (Fig. 43). The player lies face downwards, and flexes the knee strongly against the therapist's resistance; usually the therapist's hand is placed on the leg immediately above the ankle. If pain is felt in the region of the knee, the player should be asked to turn the leg inwards and outwards, with the knee flexed to 90°, against resistance. When outward rotation produces pain the biceps femoris (Fig. 43) should be palpated for tender areas; when inward rotation is painful the other hamstring muscles should be palpated.

Bursitis. Inflammation of the semimembranosus bursa is a possible cause of pain at the back of the knee. When the bursa is enlarged it

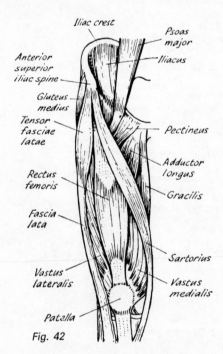

Iliac crest
Psoas major
Iliacus
Anterior superior iliac spine
Gluteus medius
Tensor fasciae latae
Pectineus
Rectus femoris
Adductor longus
Gracilis
Fascia lata
Sartorius
Vastus lateralis
Vastus medialis
Patella

Fig. 42

Front view of the muscles of the right hip and thigh.

can be located easily when the knee is extended fully; a bulge is seen at the insertion of the semimembranosus muscle. *See* Fig. 43.

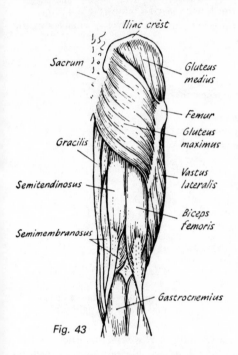

Fig. 43

Back view of the muscles of the right hip and thigh.

3: Testing the hip muscles

The hip joint lies so deep under the surrounding muscles that it is not practicable to palpate its ligaments. The ligaments are seldom involved in sports injuries, mainly because they are extremely strong and well guarded by muscles; the hip muscles, however, are frequently injured, particularly the adductor and extensor groups.

Basic anatomy

The hip muscles pass from the pelvis (the bony ring forming the lower part of the trunk) to the thigh and leg, and bring about a wide range of movement. A section of the pelvis is shown in Fig. 44; *see also* Fig. 53, p. 100.

Flexion (thigh raised forwards) is performed by the deep ilio-psoas muscle and other muscles which lie in front of the joint. (Fig. 42.) *Extension* (thigh raised backwards) is carried out by the large gluteus maximus muscle, which forms the main outline of the seat, and the hamstrings. (Fig. 43.) *Abduction* (thigh raised sideways) is brought about by the muscles lying over the outer side of the hip: gluteus medius and minimus and the tensor fasciae latae (Figs. 42 and 43). *Adduction* (thigh moved inwards) is performed by the muscles in the region of the groin. (Fig. 44.)

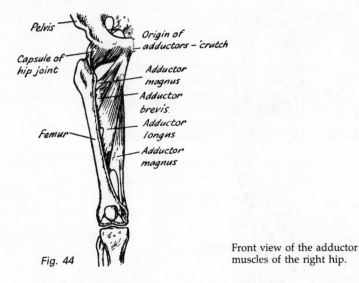

Pelvis

Capsule of hip joint

Femur

Origin of adductors – 'crutch

Adductor magnus

Adductor brevis

Adductor longus

Adductor magnus

Fig. 44

Front view of the adductor muscles of the right hip.

Inward rotation is carried out by the muscles which abduct the hip. *Outward rotation* is performed by a large number of muscles which lie at the back of the joint, especially gluteus maximus (Fig. 43); most of the adductor muscles in the groin also help in this movement.

Isolating hip movements

In testing the hip muscles it is most important that the therapist isolates the movements, and does not allow the pelvis to move. This is not easy, because normally the pelvis takes part in most of the hip movements.

The muscles are tested in the same way as the leg and thigh muscles (pp. 83 and 88). The hip movements are isolated as described below:

Abduction of right hip. The player lies on his back with the legs together. He parts the legs to the *full* extent, and then returns the right leg to its original position. The therapist places one hand on the left thigh, to keep it in position. With the other hand he gives resistance as the player abducts the right hip; the hand is placed on the outer side of the thigh, just above the knee.

Extensibility of adductors. After an injury to the *adductor* muscles full abduction of the hips (wide stride lying) is a useful test of the extensibility of the muscles.

Adduction of right hip. From the lying position the player moves the left leg inwards *as far as possible* so that it is crossed behind the right leg. The therapist places one hand on the left thigh, to keep it in position; with the other hand he gives resistance as the player adducts the right hip.

Extension of right hip. The player lies on his left side with the left thigh drawn up to the chest, the spine rounded, and the hands clasped round the knee. He extends the right hip against the therapist's resistance, being careful to keep the trunk and left thigh in their original position. During the movement it is helpful if the therapist steadies the player by supporting the lower spine with one hand.

Flexion of right hip. The player lies on his left side with the left thigh carried backwards as far as possible, and the knee flexed. He maintains this position as he flexes the right hip against the therapist's resistance; during the movement the right knee is allowed to flex.

Rotation. During hip rotation the therapist should attempt to fix the pelvis by placing the forearm across the abdomen at the level of the anterior superior iliac spines. *See* Fig. 42, p. 88. Resistance to outward and inward rotation is given by grasping the thigh firmly with the free hand.

4: Testing the spine and its muscles

Basic anatomy

The spinal column is made up of a series of joints between the bodies and arches of the vertebrae, as shown in Fig. 109, p. 171. The bodies are separated by pads of fibro-cartilage (the intervertebral discs) and bound together at the front and back by two broad, ribbon-like ligaments.

Arch joints. The joints between the vertebral arches are flat, as shown in Fig. 109, p. 171. They are strengthened by a number of powerful ligaments which pass between adjacent vertebrae.

Movements of the spine. The individual regions of the spine (lumbar, thoracic or dorsal, cervical or neck) permit different degrees of movement.

Flexion and extension are greatest in the cervical and lumbar regions. Flexion is performed by the abdominal muscles – especially the 'straight' group – and the muscles on the front of the neck. Extension is produced by the large muscle masses which lie at the back of the spine.

Lateral flexion (bending sideways) is freest in the lumbar and cervical regions. It is produced by the spinal muscles acting on one side only. In the thoracic region it is checked by the ribs.

Rotation is almost absent in the lumbar spine, but takes place freely in the cervical and thoracic regions; the range of movement is particularly good at the junction of the thoracic and lumbar vertebrae. Rotation is produced by the oblique abdominal muscles and the small muscles of the spine.

Testing the lumbar and thoracic spine

Local pain. When spinal movements produce local pain routine passive and active movements are carried out (p. 81); when the more superficial muscles and ligaments are involved an attempt is made to locate the site of the injury by palpation.

Referred pain. When spinal movements produce pain in other parts of the body the injury must be regarded as of a more serious nature. For example, if pain radiates down the back of the thigh and leg when the player flexes his hip with the knee straight, the therapist should suspect an injury to one of the lumbar intervertebral discs. Injuries of this type must be referred at once to the club doctor.

Passive tests

The player lies on a firm low couch or table. During the tests he must relax as much as possible.

Flexion. The player lies on his back and the therapist stands at the right side of the couch. He passes his right forearm behind the player's knees and lifts the thighs towards the chest, the knees being allowed to bend; the movement must be taken far enough to bring about full flexion of the hips and lumbar spine.

Extension. The player lies face downwards and the therapist stands at the right side of the couch. The therapist places his right forearm under the thighs, just above the knees, and raises the legs high enough to produce a hollowing of the lumbar spine. To prevent the upper trunk from lifting away from the couch the therapist places the palm of his left hand firmly over the lower thoracic spine.

Lateral flexion. The therapist requires an assistant for this test. The player lies on his back and the assistant places his hands on either side of the trunk, at the level of the lower ribs. The therapist stands at the right of the couch and lifts the player's legs slightly off the couch; he then carries them to the right as far as possible. During this movement the assistant exerts counter-tension, so that the side bending of the spine is confined to the lumbar region. The test is repeated to the left.

Rotation. The player lies on his back with the knees flexed to a right angle and the feet resting on the couch. The therapist stands on the right side of the couch and places the palm of his right hand over the player's left knee. He then draws the legs over to the right and downwards as much as possible (so as to produce a strong twisting movement of the lower trunk), at the same time exerting counter-tension by pressing down on the player's left shoulder with his other hand.

Active tests

The muscles are first tested by free movements; if a further test is required the therapist resists the movements. The tests are carried out with the player lying on a massage couch.

Flexion. The player raises the knees as high as possible and attempts to bring them in contact with the shoulders.

Extension. The player lies face downwards with the hands clasped behind his back. He lifts the head and shoulders as far backwards as possible.

Lateral flexion. The player lies on his left side, with his left hand resting on his right shoulder; his feet are fixed by the therapist. He raises the trunk sideways as far as possible, allowing the free hand to slide down the right leg. The test is repeated with the player lying on the right side.

Rotation. The player lies on his back with the legs well apart. He then carries the right arm across the chest and twists the trunk strongly to the left; he uses the right arm as if he were reaching for an object beyond his reach. The test is repeated to the other side.

5: Testing the wrist and its muscles

Basic anatomy

The joint is formed by the junction of three of the wrist bones (scaphoid, lunate and triquetral) with the lower end of the radius and the triangular fibro-cartilage which binds it to the ulna. (Fig. 45.)

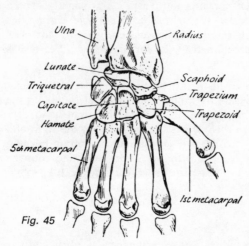

Fig. 45

Bones forming the wrist joint: back view of right wrist. The triangular fibro-cartilage has not been shown.

Ligaments. The capsular ligament surrounds the joint and is attached to the margins of the joint surfaces. It is lined by synovial membrane, and reinforced on the front and back and each side by other ligaments. Fig. 46 shows the back of the wrist.

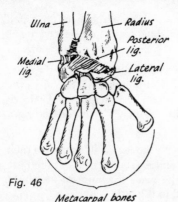

Fig. 46

Metacarpal bones

Diagrammatic impression of the ligaments of the right wrist joint: back view.

Movements. The wrist allows all movements to occur, with the exception of rotation (which takes place at the joints between the radius and ulna). The movements are produced by the forearm muscles whose tendons pass over the wrist.

Flexion is performed by muscles on the front or palmar aspect of the forearm, and *extension* by muscles on the back of the forearm. *Abduction* (moving hand sideways to thumb side of forearm) and *adduction* (opposite movement) are performed by muscles on the outer and inner sides of the forearm respectively.

Passive and active tests

The tests are carried out on the lines previously described for the joints and muscles of the lower limb, each ligament and muscle group being tested individually.

Fracture of the scaphoid. Any wrist injury which gives rise to *persistent* pain on movement of the base of the thumb, together with loss of grip, should be referred to the club doctor at once. The symptoms suggest a fracture of the scaphoid (Fig. 45, p. 94), and it is most important that this fracture should be recognized as soon as possible.

6: Testing the elbow and its muscles

Basic anatomy

The joint consists of the lower end of the humerus and the upper ends of the radius and ulna. (Fig. 47.)

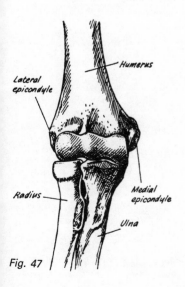

Fig. 47

Bones forming the elbow joint: front aspect of right elbow.

Ligaments. A capsular ligament surrounds the joint and is attached to the margins of the bones. It is lined by a synovial membrane, and reinforced on the inner and outer sides by two strong ligaments, the medial and lateral ligaments. (Figs. 48 and 49.)

Medial ligament. The ligament is attached to the medial or inner epicondyle of the humerus and to the inner aspect of the ulna. It is made up of three bands, as shown in Fig. 48.

Lateral ligament. This ligament is attached to the lateral or outer epicondyle of the humerus, and to the orbicular ligament which encircles the head of the radius. (Fig. 49).

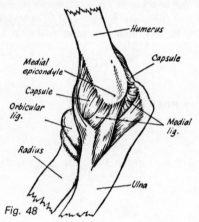

Fig. 48

Inner aspect of the right elbow joint.

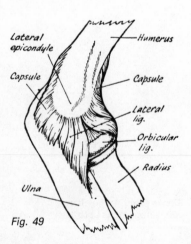

Fig. 49

Outer aspect of the right elbow joint.

Movements. These consist of hinge-like movements of flexion and extension, in which the joint is bent and stretched. *Flexion* is brought about by some of the muscles on the front of the arm, chiefly biceps, brachialis and brachio-radialis. (Fig. 54, p. 101.) *Extension* is performed by the triceps and anconeus at the back of the arm. (Fig. 55, p. 101.)

Testing the joint

Medial ligament (Fig. 48). The therapist extends the player's elbow fully, and rotates the forearm so that the palm faces forwards; he places one hand over the outer side of the arm, and the other on the inner side of the forearm, just above the wrist. He then attempts to move the forearm slightly outwards, so as to 'open up' the inner side of the joint; as he does this he must exert counter-tension on the outer side of the arm to prevent it from moving. If pain is experienced during the test the medial ligament should be palpated to find the site of the injury.

It is most important that no attempt should be made to force movement.

Lateral ligament (Fig. 49). As above, but one hand is placed over the *inner* side of the arm, and the other on the *outer* side of the forearm; the test consists of moving the forearm slightly inwards, to 'open up' the outer side of the joint.

Testing the muscles

Pain on resisted flexion of the elbow indicates an injury of one or more of the flexor muscles. Palpation is used to find the site of the injury.

A specific test for the biceps consists of the player twisting the forearm against the therapist's resistance from the palm-downward position (pronation) to the palm-upward position (supination). The test is performed with the player's elbow flexed to a right angle, and the arm kept close to the side.

Traumatic ossification. If pain is localized to the insertion area of the flexor muscles (Fig. 54, p. 101) the therapist should suspect the presence of traumatic ossification (*see* p. 191). Movement of the elbow should be prohibited, and the player referred to the club doctor.

'Tennis' and 'golf' elbow. Pain is often localized to the elbow attachments of the common wrist extensor and flexor muscles. (Figs. 131 and 132, pp. 194 and 196.) When the pain is localized to the origin of the wrist extensors it is known as 'tennis elbow'; when localized to the origin of the wrist flexors it is termed 'golfer's elbow'. For treatment *see* pp. 195 and 196.

7: Testing the shoulder and its muscles

Basic anatomy

The shoulder consists of the head of the humerus and the shallow glenoid cavity of the scapula. (Fig. 50.) It is the most unstable joint in the body, and is frequently dislocated; it relies for its stability on its muscles and not on its ligaments.

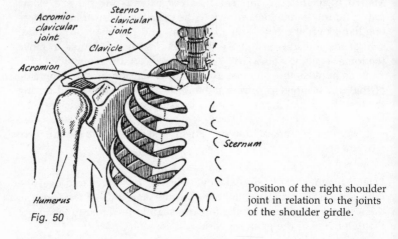

Fig. 50

Position of the right shoulder joint in relation to the joints of the shoulder girdle.

Ligaments. A capsular ligament surrounds the joint and is attached to the margins of the bones, as shown in Fig. 51. It is thin and weak, especially at the lower part, and is designed to allow a wide range of movement. The capsule is lined by a synovial membrane.

The front of the capsule is reinforced by three bands, the gleno-humeral ligaments, as shown in Fig. 51. The upper part is strengthened by the coraco-humeral ligament.

Accessory ligament. The head of the humerus is protected by the coraco-acromial ligament, which passes between the acromion and coracoid processes. (Fig. 51.)

Sub-acromial or sub-deltoid bursa. This is a large pouch of synovial membrane which exists between the deltoid and the capsule, as shown in Fig. 141, p. 204. It lies on the coraco-humeral ligament and the tendon of the supraspinatus, and under the coraco-acromial ligament. The bursa is frequently injured. *See* p. 203.

Glenoid labrum or lip. This is a rim of fibro-cartilage which is attached round the margin of the glenoid cavity; it deepens the cavity and protects the edge of the bone.

Rotator cuff. The cuff consists of an important group of muscles which strengthen the capsule on various aspects, and blend with it. The muscles are: subscapularis on the front; supraspinatus above; and infraspinatus and teres minor at the back. (Figs. 52 and 53. *See* also p. 204.)

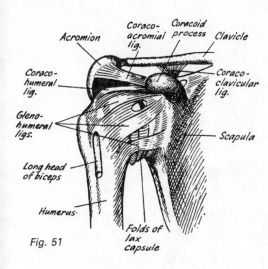

Fig. 51

Front view of the right shoulder joint.

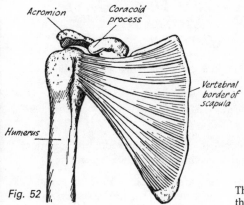

Fig. 52

The subscapularis muscle of the right shoulder joint.

Movement of the shoulder

The shoulder is a ball-and-socket joint, and capable of all movements. It moves in conjunction with the joints of the shoulder girdle: the acromio-clavicular and sterno-clavicular joints. (Fig. 50, p. 98.)

Flexion (arm carried forward) is brought about mainly by the pectoralis major and the front fibres of the deltoid. (Fig. 54.)

Extension (arm carried backward) is produced by the back fibres of deltoid, the teres major and latissimus dorsi. (Figs. 53 and 55.)

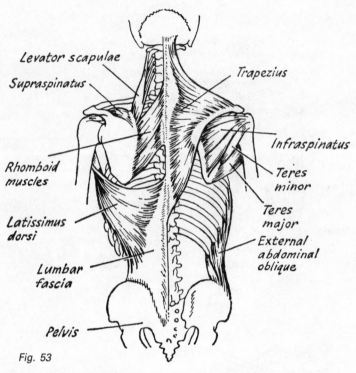

Fig. 53

Back view of the trunk showing some of the main muscles of the shoulder joint and shoulder girdle.

Abduction (arm raised sideways) is performed chiefly by the deltoid. (Fig. 54.)

Adduction (opposite movement to abduction) is brought about mainly by the pectoralis major and latissimus dorsi. (Figs. 53 and 54.)

Outward rotation (arm turned outwards so that palm faces forwards) is performed by the back fibres of the deltoid, the infraspinatus and teres minor. (Fig. 55.)

Inward rotation (opposite movement to outward rotation) is produced mainly by the pectoralis major, the subscapularis, latissimus dorsi, teres major and the front fibres of deltoid. (Figs. 52 to 54.)

Retraction. From a position where the arm is held forwards at right angles to the trunk, the arm is moved *horizontally* backwards until it is held sideways in line with the trunk. The movement is brought about by the latissimus dorsi, teres major, the back fibres of deltoid, and other outward rotator muscles. (Figs. 53 and 55.)

Protraction (opposite movement to retraction) is produced by the pectoralis major, subscapularis, and the front fibres of deltoid. (Figs. 52 and 54.)

Circumduction. A combination of the previous movements; the arm is moved in a circular fashion.

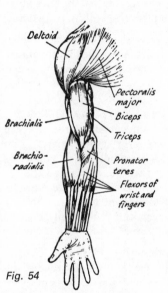

Fig. 54

Front view of the superficial muscles of the right arm and forearm.

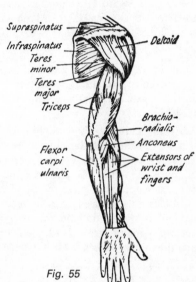

Fig. 55

Back view of the superficial muscles of the right arm and forearm. The trapezius muscle, which covers the back of the neck and shoulder, has not been shown.

Structures injured

The ligaments of the shoulder are not often injured in a direct manner, because their laxity saves them from being stretched unduly. The other structures of the joint, particularly the muscles and tendons, are frequently injured. Because of their complex arrangement it is often necessary to localize the site of the injury accurately, and specific tests are of great value.

Testing the muscles

The tests given here cover the main muscles of the shoulder.

Abductor muscles. Pain experienced when the player abducts the shoulder freely or against the therapist's resistance indicates an injury of the deltoid or the tendon of the supraspinatus. (Figs. 53 and 54, pp. 100 and 101.)

Testing the deltoid. The player raises the arm sideways to shoulder height. *Keeping the arm at this level* he moves it against the therapist's resistance: (*a*) forwards through 90° (protraction), (*b*) backwards to the sideways stretch position (retraction), and (*c*) backwards as far as possible.

Pain on forward movement indicates that the front fibres of deltoid are involved; pain on backward movement suggests that the back fibres of the muscle are injured. The area of injury is sought by palpation.

Testing the supraspinatus tendon. If the forward and backward movements of the arm do not give rise to pain, it is probable that the injury is localized to the tendon of the supraspinatus. The tendon is palpated on the upper part of the greater tuberosity of the humerus. *See* Fig. 53, p. 100.

Adductor muscles. Pain experienced when the player adducts the shoulder against the therapist's resistance (movement starts with arm sideways at shoulder level and ends with arm at side) indicates an injury of one of the four adductor muscles: pectoralis major, latissimus dorsi, teres major or teres minor. (Figs. 53 and 54, pp. 100 and 101.)

To locate the injured area the test used for the deltoid (*see* previous section) is repeated. Pain on forward movement indicates that the pectoralis major is involved. Pain on backward movement suggests that the injury is localized to the latissimus dorsi, teres major or minor.

Testing latissimus dorsi and teres major. Both these muscles help to rotate the shoulder inwards. To test them the player inwardly rotates the shoulder against the therapist's resistance, with the elbow bent to 90° and the arm kept to the side. The movement is taken as far as possible, the therapist resisting at the forearm, just above the wrist.

If pain occurs during this test the therapist should palpate the latissimus dorsi and teres major to locate the site of the injury.

Testing teres minor. This muscle helps to rotate the shoulder outwards. The previous test is repeated, but the shoulder is rotated *outwards* as far as possible. If pain occurs during the test the therapist should attempt to palpate the teres minor.

Outward rotator muscles. To test these muscles the player outwardly rotates the shoulder against resistance with the elbow bent to 90° and the arm kept to the side. The movement is taken to the full extent, the therapist resisting at the forearm.

Pain produced by resisted outward rotation indicates an injury of either the infraspinatus or teres minor, generally at the insertion point of the tendon.

To differentiate between the actions of the two muscles the following tests are made:

1. The player attempts to raise the arm sideways against the therapist's resistance. If pain is experienced during this test the injury can be regarded as being localized to the infraspinatus, because the muscle assists in abducting the shoulder in addition to being an outward rotator.

2. The player attempts to adduct the shoulder by pressing the arm strongly against his side. Pain experienced during this test indicates an injury of the teres minor, because the muscle assists in adducting the shoulder in addition to being an outward rotator.

Palpation. When the tests have been carried out the therapist palpates the affected muscle and tendon to locate the exact area of injury.

Note. In testing the outward rotators it must be remembered that the back fibres of the deltoid assist in outward rotation movements. For deltoid test *see* p. 100.

Inward rotator muscles. The muscles are tested in the same way as the outward rotators, with the exception that the shoulder joint is rotated inwards until the forearm touches the chest.

Pain produced by resisted inward rotation indicates an injury of one of the following muscles: subscapularis, pectoralis major, latissimus dorsi or teres major.

To differentiate between the actions of the muscles the player raises his arm sideways to shoulder height. *Keeping it at this level* he moves it against the therapist's resistance (*a*) forwards through 90°, and (*b*) backwards as far as possible.

Pain on forward movement indicates that the pectoralis major or subscapularis is injured; pain on backward movement suggests that the injury is localized to latissimus dorsi or teres major.

Pectoralis major or subscapularis. The pectoralis major is an adductor of the shoulder, while the subscapularis is an inward rotator only. To distinguish between the actions of the two muscles the player adducts the shoulder by pressing the arm strongly against his side. If the pectoral muscle is involved the area of injury is found by palpation.

Latissimus dorsi or teres major. Both muscles have similar actions, and so the injury must be localized by careful palpation.

Testing the sub-acromial (sub-deltoid) bursa

Sub-acromial or sub-deltoid bursitis is frequently the cause of pain in the shoulder joint. Generally most pain is experienced on resisted abduction, because of the contraction of the deltoid.

The bursa (Fig. 141, p. 204) can be palpated if the shoulder is first adducted, so that the arm rests across the chest. The therapist's fingers are placed on the upper part of the shoulder in the vicinity of the acromion process. For treatment *see* p. 204.

Part 3

Treatment of lower limb injuries

Chapter 7
Injuries of the foot

Foot strain

Foot strain is a subacute or chronic strain of the tarsal ligaments (Fig. 56). It is not a common condition in sport, but it occurs from time to time and is not always easy to clear up.

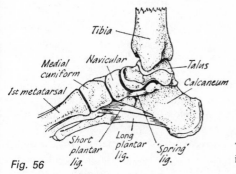

Fig. 56

Three of the tarsal ligaments: inner aspect of right foot.

Causes. Foot strain may be caused by persistent over-use of the feet and by a rapid increase in body-weight. It sometimes occurs after a fracture of the leg when the supporting plaster cast has been removed.

Symptoms. Pain is the chief symptom. At first it is localized to the inner border of the foot, and is only felt when the player is tired. Later it becomes more constant, is aggravated by weight-bearing, and often radiates over the foot and calf. There may be some swelling of the foot and ankle, which gets worse towards the end of the day.

When the foot is examined there is usually tenderness on pressure over the inner border. If the foot is moved passively there is limitation of movement in at least one direction, and pain at the extreme of that movement.

Treatment. The player must endeavour to relieve the strained ligaments of tension by restricting his activities for a few weeks, and

paying particular attention to the position of his feet when standing.
The feet should point forwards and be placed about 2 in. apart. The
legs should be braced firmly so that the knee caps face directly forwards
and do not 'squint' inwards; a small degree of outward rotation of the
hips is essential to counteract any tendency to 'squinting' knees. The
body-weight should be taken by the heels and the heads of the 1st
and 5th metatarsal bones; the toes should be kept straight with the
pads pressed down against the shoes.

Massage and exercises. Massage of the foot and leg is helpful. Simple
exercises to mobilize the stiff joints of the foot should be practised
daily. For example, sitting with one knee crossed over the other: (*a*)
foot turning inwards and outwards, (*b*) ankle bending and stretching,
and (*c*) foot circling. If the joints are very stiff the foot may have to be
manipulated by a surgeon. A general anaesthetic is used, and the foot
moved into full inversion and eversion, plantar- and dorsiflexion.
After-treatment consists of massage and exercises.

Metatarsalgia
('Dropped' transverse arch)

Metatarsalgia consists of pain beneath the forefoot in the region of the
metatarsal heads. The pain is experienced on weight-bearing, and
when pressure is exerted on the metatarsal heads during examination
of the foot.

The condition is caused by a weakness of the small intrinsic muscles
of the foot which normally bind the metatarsal bones together and
maintain them in an arched position. The heads are allowed to splay
out, and too much pressure falls on them in weight-bearing. The
excessive pressure may lead to the formation of callosities beneath the
points of pressure.

Weakness of the intrinsic muscles results from over-use of the foot;
it may also occur when a fracture of the leg is immobilized in a plaster
cast for several weeks. Fractures of the metatarsal bones also cause
weakness of the intrinsic muscles.

Treatment. The intrinsic muscles must be strengthened by special foot
exercises; faradic stimulation by means of faradic baths is also very
helpful. The use of a felt metatarsal pad (Fig. 59) for a period of 2 to
3 weeks is of value in preventing pain while weight-bearing.

Intrinsic exercises. (1) Sitting, shortening of each foot in turn (flexion of
the metatarso-phalangeal joints with toes kept straight), as shown in
Fig. 57. (2) Sitting, with feet on floor in tray of sand, attempting to
part and close the toes. (3) Sitting, with toes resting on a book, flexion

of the metatarso-phalangeal joints with toes kept straight (Fig. 58): each foot is exercised in turn.

Metatarsal pad. A shield-shaped pad is cut from adhesive felt, ¼ to ⅜ in. thick; it measures approximately 4 in. in length and 3 in. at its

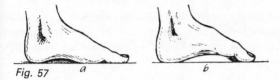

Fig. 57   *a*   *b*

Foot shortening: an exercise to strengthen the small intrinsic muscles.

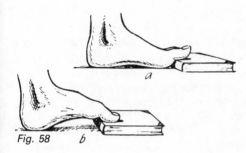

Fig. 58   *b*

A more difficult exercise for the intrinsic muscles.

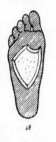 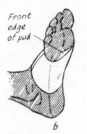

Front edge of pad

a   *b*

Fig. 59

a. Adhesive felt pad fitted behind metatarsal heads.
b. Two turns of elastoplast are taken round the forefoot over the pad.

widest point. When the pad has been cut the edges on the non-adhesive side are bevelled with scissors.

The pad is fitted just behind the metatarsal heads, as shown in Fig. 59a. A couple of turns of 3 in. elastoplast are then taken round the forefoot over the pad, as shown in Fig. 59b. The strapping prevents the pad from shifting backwards when the foot is used for weight-bearing; it also acts as a brace for the metatarsal bones.

Morton's metatarsalgia

This condition is characterized by metatarsal pain combined with a *radiating* pain in the 3rd and 4th toes. It is caused by a fibrous thickening or 'neuroma' of the digital nerve of the cleft between the 3rd and 4th metatarsal bones. The cause of the thickening is uncertain.

Treatment. The club doctor usually suggests the wearing of a metatarsal pad, as previously described. If this fails to relieve the symptoms surgical treatment is usually recommended; the thickened segment of the nerve is removed.

Hallux rigidus

Hallux rigidus is the term used to describe a gradual stiffening of the metatarso-phalangeal joint of the big toe. The condition is fairly common in footballers, and is caused by repeated 'stubbing' of the toe and similar minor injuries.

Osteo-arthritic changes occur in the joint, and the player complains *at times* of pain in the base of the big toe when walking. The push-off movement of the foot is the main source of trouble, because of the limited amount of extension in the joint.

Treatment. In the majority of cases treatment is not required. When the joint is irritated by a strain or a knock, however, a course of short-wave diathermy helps to relieve the pain.

If the joint becomes extremely stiff and painful the player should be seen by an orthopaedic surgeon. He may advise the fitting of a 'rocker bar' to the sole of the shoe (in order to replace the movement of the joint), or an operation to create a mobile, painless joint.

Plantar fasciitis

Plantar fasciitis is a common complaint. It is characterized by pain and tenderness beneath the front part of the heel on standing and walking, and is thought to be an inflammation of the plantar fascia and the short muscles at their attachment to the heel bone. The inflammation may be due to injury or a septic focus, e.g. infection of the teeth or tonsils.

Treatment. The heel should be cushioned by a sponge-rubber pad which is cut to fit the back part of the shoe and hollowed out exactly opposite the tender area. Short-wave diathermy should be used.

Many cases of plantar fasciitis are very resistant to treatment, and may take weeks to clear up. The player should be advised to rest as much as possible.

Tender heel pad

Pain felt behind the hind part of the heel on standing and walking is a condition which sometimes troubles sportsmen. The site of the tenderness is the fibro-fatty tissue beneath the weight-bearing area of the heel bone. In the majority of cases the injury is a simple bruising; in other cases there is no history of injury and the condition seems to be a mild inflammation.

Treatment. Generally the condition improves slowly without treatment. Recovery is aided by cushioning the heel with a piece of sponge-rubber, which is placed inside the shoe, and by treating the tender area with short-wave diathermy.

Chapter 8

Injuries of the ankle ligaments

Sprain: general considerations. The term 'sprain' is defined here, because considerable confusion exists as to its exact meaning.

Normally the muscles protect the joints and prevent their ligaments from being injured. During a sudden, unexpected movement the muscles may be momentarily 'off guard'; the ligaments are then exposed to the full force of the movement, and are either stretched unduly or 'sprained', or torn completely.

Degrees of sprain. Sprains may be divided into: *1st degree* or minor sprains, when a few fibres of a ligament are torn, and *2nd degree* sprains, when a greater number of fibres are torn. In both types of injury the stability of the joint is not impaired.

Complete tear of ligament. When a ligament is stretched so violently that it is completely ruptured the injury must not be regarded as a sprain, but as a potential subluxation or dislocation. Such an injury is serious; if it is not recognized and treated by immobilization it leads to an unstable joint which is constantly 'giving way'.

Sprains

The front and middle bands of the lateral ligament of the ankle are frequently sprained (Fig. 60). The same bands of the medial ligament (Fig. 36, p. 83) are also sometimes sprained. Sprains of both ligaments

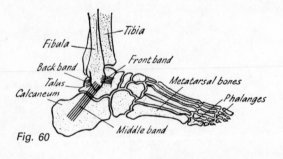

Fig. 60

Diagram of the lateral ligament of the right ankle joint.

are often associated with a sprain of the front part of the capsule.

The lateral ligament is sprained by any twist or turn of the foot which forces it down into plantar-flexion and inwards into inversion. The medial ligament is injured in the same way, but the foot is forced into eversion and plantar-flexion.

Complete rupture of lateral ligament

Complete rupture of the lateral ligament is not an uncommon injury. It is caused by a violent inversion strain, the front and middle bands of the ligament being torn away from the lateral malleolus. This allows the talus to tilt in the mortice of the ankle, making the joint most insecure.

Sprain of lateral ligament
1st degree or minor sprain

Main symptoms: Small amount of swelling, some pain, and slight loss of function.

Treatment: immediately after injury

Strips of white lint soaked in lead lotion are placed round the injured joint: a 3 or 4 in. crêpe bandage is then applied in a modified figure-of-eight manner (Fig. 69, p. 117), as described below. The player is allowed to walk, but should limit his activities as much as possible for 24 hours.

Bandaging: position of foot

The bandage is applied with the player in the half-lying position on a massage couch; a pillow is placed lengthwise under the injured limb. (Fig. 61.) Throughout the major part of the bandaging the foot must be held in an upward and outward direction (dorsiflexion combined with eversion), so that the finished bandage will tend to keep the injured ligament in a shortened position and prevent it from being stretched.

The therapist holds the foot in one hand and the bandage in the other; he has to change the position of the hands frequently, but he must not allow the corrected position of the foot to alter appreciably.

The bandage is applied reasonably tightly, a firm degree of tension being exerted on each turn as it is carried round the limb.

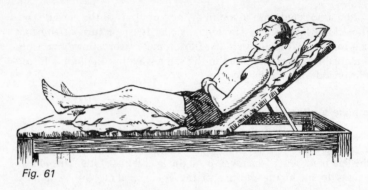

Fig. 61

Half-lying. The pillow support for the leg and thigh allows the ankle to be bandaged or strapped without difficulty.

Modified figure-of-eight bandage

1. The free end of the bandage is placed on the outer border of the foot, so that the front edge is just behind the head of the 5th metatarsal bone. The bandage is then passed across the top of the foot, the front edge being kept behind the head of the 1st metatarsal; it is then carried under the sole and back to the starting position; this turn is repeated. (Fig. 62.)

2. The therapist presses the foot upwards and outwards with one hand; with the other he carries the bandage upwards in a slanting direction across the top of the foot to the inner border. The bandage is then passed straight under the foot to the outer border.

3. The bandage is carried downwards in a slanting direction across the foot to the inner border, so that it crosses the previous turn. It is then passed under the foot to the outer border. (Fig. 63.)

4. The bandage is passed in a slanting direction across the top of the foot, and round the inner side of the ankle. It is then taken behind the ankle to the outer side. (Fig. 64.)

5. The bandage is carried over the lateral malleolus and then passed downwards in a slanting direction across the top of the foot to the inner border, so that it crosses the previous turn; it is then taken under the foot to the outer border. (Fig. 65.)

6. The bandage is carried across the previous turn in a slanting direction to the upper part of the medial malleolus (*see* Fig. 67). It is then taken behind the leg, so that the lower border is immediately behind the lateral malleolus. (Fig. 66.)

7. The bandage is carried across the front of the ankle to the inner side of the heel; it passes over the medial malleolus and covers the whole of the inner surface of the heel. (Fig. 67.)

8. The bandage is taken round the heel to the outer side, and carried upwards in a slanting direction to the front of the leg; it covers the

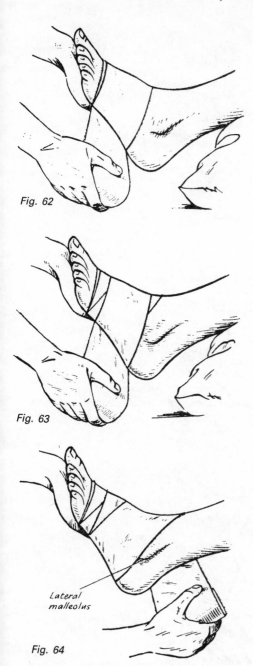

Fig. 62

Fig. 63

Lateral
malleolus

Fig. 64

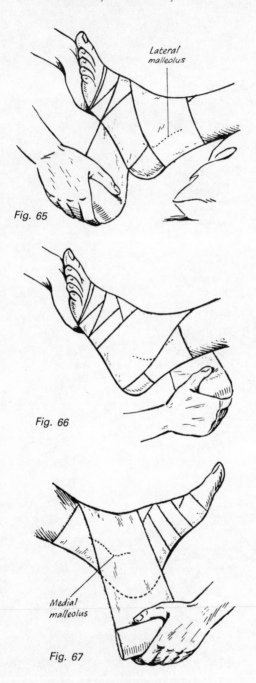

Fig. 65

Fig. 66

Fig. 67

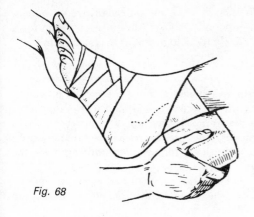

Figs. 62–68. Supporting the ankle with a crêpe bandage after a minor sprain of the lateral ligament. Before the bandage is applied, strips of lint soaked in lead lotion are placed round the joint; they are not shown here.

Fig. 68

outer surface of the heel completely, and passes over the lateral malleolus. Next, the bandage is passed across the inner side of the leg in an upward slanting direction; it is then carried round the leg to the outer side. Fig. 68.

9. Several turns of bandage are taken round the leg, the finish being made at the outer side. The bandage is then pinned off. Fig. 69 shows the completed bandage.

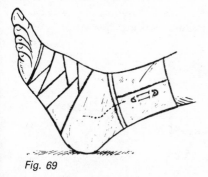

Fig. 69   The completed crêpe bandage.

Treatment: 24 hours after injury
(For period of about 1 week)

Physiotherapy. The bandage and lint strips are removed. Short-wave diathermy, massage and foot and ankle exercises are given daily. Strengthening exercises for the evertor muscles are most important. *Examples*: (*a*) From the half-lying position (Fig. 61, p. 114) the player turns the injured foot outwards as much as possible, 'holds' the final position for a moment, and then allows the foot to return to its former place. (*b*) From sitting the player raises the outer borders of the feet from the floor as much as possible, 'holds' the raised position for a moment, and then allows the borders to return to the floor again. Both exercises must be performed fairly slowly.

Strapping. After treatment a C-shaped pad of adhesive felt is centred over the lateral ligament, and the ankle is strapped with 3 in. elastoplast. (Fig. 70.) When the player moves the ankle and foot the pressure of the pad against the moving structures exerts a massaging effect on the ligament; this helps to disperse the swelling and improves the blood supply of the injured part.

The pad is about 4 in. × 2 in., and is cut from a piece of adhesive felt, 3/16 in. or 1/4 in. thick. The edges of the non-adhesive side are bevelled with scissors, so that the pad fits snugly under the strapping. (Fig. 70.)

In applying the strapping the same figure-of-eight bandaging technique is used as previously described, with the exception that only one turn of elastoplast is required when the strapping is started, and the finish consists of two turns instead of several. A strip of zinc oxide plaster is usually stuck over the cut end of the strapping, to prevent it from wrinkling up. (Fig. 70.)

Resuming training. When the player can use the ankle normally the lateral ligament is tested passively (p. 82); if the result is satisfactory training is resumed. At each training session the ankle must be

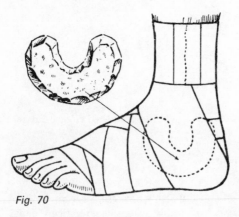

Strapping for auto-massage. A C-shaped pad of adhesive felt is placed over the lateral ligament and the ankle strapped with elastoplast.

Fig. 70

supported by a reinforced elastoplast strapping (Fig. 78, p. 122); the same type of strapping should be used when the player returns to the game. *See* p. 22.

Reinforced elastoplast strapping

The ankle is strapped with 3 in. elastoplast, the figure-of-eight bandaging technique described on p. 114 being used; fewer turns are used, however, because the finished strapping is strengthened by the addition of three strips of 2 in. zinc oxide adhesive plaster. One of the strips has a deep V-shaped notch cut in one of its borders at the central point.

Strapping technique. The strips of zinc oxide strapping are applied with the player's hip and knee flexed, and the ball of the foot resting against the therapist's chest, as shown in Fig. 71. Throughout the strapping the therapist presses the foot strongly into an upward and outward direction with his chest, the player preventing the limb from being pushed up by resisting with his knee and hip muscles. This technique allows the therapist to use both hands in strapping, while the foot is kept in a corrected position.

The cut lengths of strapping must be close at hand. They may hang from the edge of a table placed near to the therapist, or from the massage couch, as shown in Fig. 71.

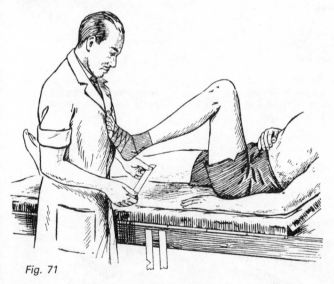

Fig. 71

Reinforced elastoplast strapping for ankle. Method of supporting foot while applying strips of zinc oxide adhesive plaster over elastoplast support.

Application of 1st (stirrup) strap

The therapist corrects the position of the foot with his chest; he then takes the two ends of the first strap in his hands and places the centre

of the strap on the under surface of the heel, as shown in Fig. 72. He
carries the inner end of the strap up the inner side of the leg, so that
it covers the medial malleolus. (Fig. 73.) Next, he takes the outer end
of the strap up the outer side of the leg in the same way, the front
part of the lateral malleolus being covered to a greater extent than the
back part. (Fig. 74.) He then moulds the strap closely to the elastoplast
strapping by running his hands smoothly up and down the leg and
heel.

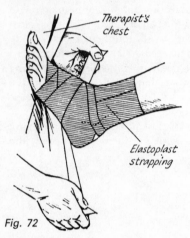

Fig. 72

Positioning the stirrup strap
under the heel while the foot
is pressed in an upward and
outward direction by the
therapist's chest.

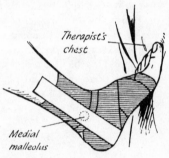

Fig. 73

The inner end of the stirrup
strap covers the medial
malleolus.

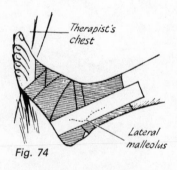

Fig. 74

The outer end of the stirrup
strap in position.

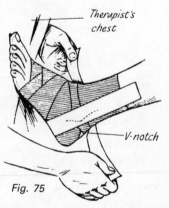

Fig. 75

The notched strap is placed
at the back of the ankle, with
the notch centred over the
Achilles tendon.

Application of 2nd (notched) strap

The notched strap is applied over the stirrup strap. It is placed at the back of the ankle, at the level of the malleoli, so that the notch is centred over the Achilles tendon. (Fig. 75.) The outer end of the strap is then passed downwards and inwards over the foot in a slanting direction; the inner end of the strap is taken downwards and outwards in the same way, so that the two ends cross in front of the ankle, as shown in Fig. 76.

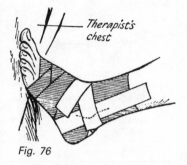

Therapist's chest

Fig. 76

The notched strap in position.

It is most important that each end of the strap should be moulded separately over the elastoplast strapping; on no account should the therapist pull on both ends at once. This also applies to the application of the third strap.

Application of 3rd (cross) strap

The strap is applied under the foot in front of the ankle, as shown in Fig. 77. The inner end is taken in an upward and outward direction across the front of the ankle. The outer end of the strap is then passed upwards and inwards across the front of the ankle, so that it crosses the other end. (Fig. 78.)

Sprain of lateral ligament
2nd degree or severe sprain

Main symptoms: Moderate amount of swelling; considerable pain and loss of function.

The injury should be seen by the club doctor as soon as possible.

Treatment: immediately after injury

Support. Two forms of treatment may be used. (1) A pressure bandage (Fig. 89, p. 127) is applied, as described here, and the foot and ankle

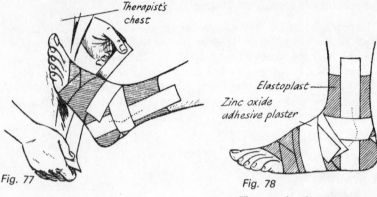

Fig. 77

Positioning the cross strap under the foot.

Fig. 78

The completed strapping. After a sprain of the ankle this type of support is used at each training session and when the player returns to the game or event.

are immersed for about 10 minutes in a deep bowl or pail of ice-cold water (p. 24); the bandage is then removed and another pressure bandage applied. (2) Strips of white lint soaked in lead lotion are placed round the ankle; a pressure bandage is then applied.

Rest and elevation. The player should not take weight on the injured leg for at least 24 hours; when he stands or walks he must use elbow crutches. He should go to bed as soon as possible and rest with the injured leg elevated on pillows, so that the foot is higher than the hip. He should be instructed to loosen the bandage if the swelling increases and the bandage causes pain.

Pressure bandage

Four rectangular-shaped pieces of cotton wool are applied to the ankle and foot, each piece being compressed by turns of calico bandage. A figure-of-eight bandaging technique is used.

Each piece of cotton wool should be about 13 in. wide and long enough to be wrapped round the ankle with an overlap of a few inches: 20 in. is an approximate length. Two calico bandages are needed, each 6 yds. × 4 in.; their ends are sewn together to make one long bandage. Calico bandages can be made up from a length of calico 6 yds. × 36 in. The bandage widths are marked off with scissor cuts at one end; the strips are then torn in a lengthwise direction.

Position of foot. The bandage is applied with the player in half-lying, a pillow being arranged lengthwise under the thigh and leg, as shown in Fig. 61, p. 114. The four pieces of cotton wool are placed on the player's thigh, so that the therapist can reach them easily when he is bandaging the ankle.

During the major part of the bandaging the foot must be held in an upward and outward direction by one of the therapist's hands, while the bandage is held by the other. The position of the hands has to be changed frequently.

Technique and precautions. The bandage is applied tightly, the tension being increased as each layer of wool is added. When the bandage has been finished the circulation of the leg must be checked to see if it has been impaired. The toes should be pinched, to see if the colour returns quickly to the skin in the normal way. If it does not it is an indication that the deep circulation is restricted, and the bandage must be removed immediately. The appearance of the veins of the toes must be observed carefully; if they are distended and the skin has taken on a purple tinge, it is an indication that the bandage is restricting the superficial circulation, and it must be taken off. The sound limb should always be used as a comparison.

Application of 1st piece of wool

1. The first piece of cotton wool is placed under the player's heel, so that the heel rests in the centre. (Fig. 79.) The wool is wrapped round the foot and ankle, so that the edges overlap.

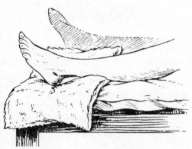

Pressure bandage. The heel rests in the middle of the first piece of cotton wool.

Fig. 79

2. The end of the bandage is placed on the outer border of the foot, over the wool, so that the front edge is immediately behind the head of the 5th metatarsal bone. The bandage is then taken round the foot twice, to secure the end. (Fig. 80.)

3. The therapist presses the foot in an upward and outward direction with one hand; with the other he carries the bandage upward in a sloping direction to the inner aspect of the heel. He then takes the bandage round the heel to the outer side. (Fig.81.)

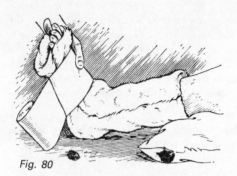

Fig. 80

Outer aspect of ankle: the start of the bandaging.

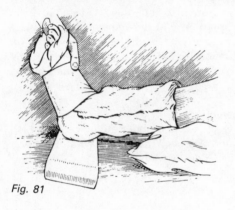

Fig. 81

The foot is pressed upwards and outwards as the bandage is taken round the heel.

4. The therapist carries the bandage downwards and inwards in a sloping direction across the top of the foot to the inner border, so that the outer side of the ankle is covered. It is then passed under the foot to the outer border. (Fig. 82.)

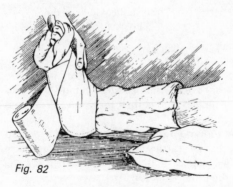

Fig. 82

The first figure-of-eight turn has been completed.

5. The bandaging is continued in this manner, the turns gradually covering the foot and extending above the ankle. Fig. 83 shows the bandage when the first layer of wool has been covered. Note the free edges of wool at the upper and lower limits of the bandage.

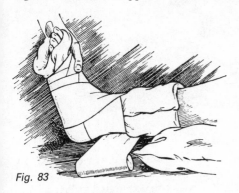

Fig. 83

Extent of bandage cover for first piece of cotton wool.

Application of 2nd piece of wool

1. One end of the second piece of wool is tucked well in between the free strip of bandage and the first piece of cotton wool. The wool is moulded round the foot and ankle, so that the loose end lies behind the free part of the bandage. (Fig. 84.)

2. A horizontal turn of bandage is taken round the leg, over the new piece of wool.

3. Figure-of-eight turns of bandage are taken over the wool until it is covered (Fig. 85), the technique being similar to that previously described for covering the first layer.

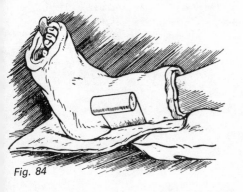

Fig. 84

Outer aspect of ankle: the second piece of wool has been added.

Application of 3rd piece of wool

The third piece of wool is added to the bandage in the same way as the second piece. It is covered by figure-of-eight turns of bandage, the free edges being left uncovered.

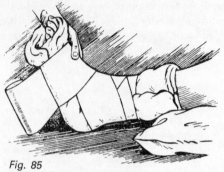

Fig. 85

The covering of the second piece of wool has been completed.

Application of 4th piece of wool

1. The fourth piece of wool is added in the same way as the second piece (*see* Fig. 84). The upper edges of the four layers of wool are then turned over to a depth of about 3 in., as demonstrated in Fig. 86. Two turns of bandage are taken round them. (Fig. 87.)

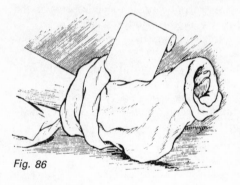

Fig. 86

Inner aspect of ankle: the *fourth* piece of cotton wool has been added. The upper edges of the four layers of wool have been turned over.

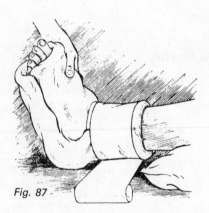

Fig. 87

Outer aspect of ankle showing firm upper border of bandage.

2. The foot and ankle are then bandaged as before until the fourth piece of wool is covered. (Fig. 88.)

3. The lower edges of the four layers of wool are then turned over, and bound down by two turns of bandage.

4. The remaining length of bandage is used up by being taken round the foot and ankle in figure-of-eight turns. The bandage is completed by two horizontal turns being made round the leg. (Fig. 89.)

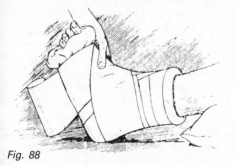

The fourth piece of cotton wool has been covered. Note the free margin of wool above the toes.

Fig. 88

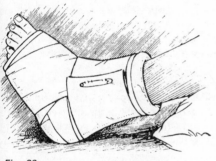

The completed pressure bandage.

Fig. 89

Treatment: 24 hours after injury

Physiotherapy. The pressure bandage is removed. One of the following treatments is then given: interferential therapy (using plate electrodes), ultrasound, or short-wave diathermy (using inducto-thermy cable). Contrast baths may also be used.

The player is encouraged to exercise the foot and ankle within a pain-free range of movement while he rests with the leg elevated; eversion movements should be emphasized (p. 117). Weight-bearing exercises are not allowed.

Support. If the ankle is badly swollen it is best to reapply the pressure bandage and advise the player to rest for a further 24 hours. If the original swelling is considerably reduced, however, the ankle should be supported by a reinforced elastoplast strapping, as described on p. 116, and the player encouraged to walk as normally as possible; a stick may be necessary at first. He should be warned not to stand or walk too much; when sitting he should have the injured foot elevated on a stool.

Treatment: 48 hours after injury
(For period of 2 to 3 weeks)

Physiotherapy. The pressure bandage or strapping is removed. Interferential therapy (using plate electrodes), ultrasound, or short-wave diathermy (using inductothermy cable) is given. This is followed by massage – including frictions to the lateral ligament – and non-weight-bearing exercises within the limit of pain. *Examples*. Half-lying (Fig. 61, p. 114): (a) turning each foot outwards in turn, (b) bending (dorsiflexing) each ankle in turn, (c) bending and stretching the ankles alternately, and (d) turning the feet alternately inwards and outwards. Sitting: (a) raising the outer borders of the feet from the floor, and (b) bending each ankle in turn.

Support. After treatment the ankle is supported by a reinforced elastoplast strapping (p. 116). Training in walking is important; emphasis must be laid on taking even steps, putting full weight on the injured foot, and using the ankle normally. Generally a stick is not necessary.

Progressing treatment. Interferential or ultrasonic therapy is discontinued when the swelling subsides. Heat therapy, transverse frictions and exercises are continued. The exercises must be progressed gradually in strength and mobility, and should include partial and full weight-bearing movements and resisted movements.

Strengthening exercises. (a) Heel raising, using the arms to take some of the body-weight (Fig. 11, p. 47). (b) Heel raising, but the arms hang to the sides and do not assist the movement. (c) The player lies on his uninjured side on a massage couch, with a pillow placed between his legs and feet. He turns the injured foot outwards (eversion) either freely or against a weight resistance. (d) The player everts the injured foot against the resistance of a simple weight-and-pulley circuit.

Mobility exercises. (a) The player takes the half-lying position on a massage couch (Fig. 61, p. 114) with his feet over the end. He points *both* feet to the left and right alternately in a continuous rhythmical manner. (b) Position as previous exercise, but the player circles the injured foot downwards, outwards, upwards and inwards. The movement should be performed in a smooth continuous manner; the outward (eversion) movement must be emphasized. In both exercises it is essential for the player to keep the legs still, and to restrict the movements to the foot and ankle.

Resuming training. At the end of two to three weeks' treatment the lateral ligament is tested passively (p. 82); if the result is satisfactory, training is resumed; at each training session the ankle must be supported by a reinforced elastoplast strapping (p. 116). The same type of strapping should be used when the player returns to the game. *See* p. 22.

Complete tear of lateral ligament

Main symptoms: Large amount of swelling, which occurs rapidly, and considerable pain; gross loss of function. During inversion movements of the foot there is excessive mobility of the talus (Fig. 35, p. 83), which is no longer held firmly in the mortice of the ankle joint.

The player must be seen by the club doctor as soon as possible. The ankle will be X-rayed with the foot inverted to check up on the position of the talus.

Treatment

Immobilization in plaster cast. The torn ligament will repair itself if the ankle is immobilized in a plaster-of-paris cast for a period of 8 to 10 weeks. The cast extends from the webs of the toes to just below the knee, with the foot fixed at a right angle to the leg.

When the cast is dry the player is allowed to take weight on the injured foot, and it is most important that he is taught to walk as normally as possible. A leather overshoe with a rocker sole is worn over the foot. It may be necessary for the player to use two sticks when he first starts to walk.

Exercise therapy. During the period in plaster the player should practise exercises to maintain the strength of the leg muscles. For example: (*a*) strong bending of the toes and slow recoil, (*b*) strong stretching of the toes and slow recoil, (*c*) 'attempted' foot eversion, and (*d*) 'attempted' ankle bending and stretching. He should also exercise the knee and hip muscles. *See also* Chapter 17, p. 209.

Plaster cast removed. When the cast is removed exercises are used to strengthen the leg muscles and restore the mobility of the ankle and foot joints. Care must be taken to graduate the exercises carefully. Non-weight-bearing exercises are used at first, and progressed to resisted and weight-bearing exercises. *See* p. 210. Special attention should be paid to strengthening the evertor muscles.

Dispersing swelling. Daily massage of the leg, ankle and foot is of value in improving the circulation and dispersing any oedema or swelling. Swelling of the ankle and foot tends to occur when the plaster is removed, because the walls of the capillary blood vessels have lost their tone; as a result the plasma or blood fluid leaks into the tissue spaces.

Support. To prevent swelling a crêpe bandage should be worn for about 2 weeks after the plaster cast is removed. It is applied as described below, and must extend from the webs of the toes to the tibial tubercle. (Fig. 90, p. 131.) The player should remove the bandage at night when he goes to bed, and reapply it in the morning before he gets up.

Resuming training. About 3 to 4 weeks after the removal of the plaster the lateral ligament is tested passively, as described on p. 82; if the result is satisfactory training is started. At each training session the ankle must be supported by a reinforced elastoplast strapping (p. 116). The ankle must be strapped in the same way when the player returns to the game. *See* p. 22.

Crêpe bandage support for foot and leg

A 4 in. crêpe bandage is used. It is applied reasonably tightly, a firm degree of tension being exerted on each turn. The half-lying position is used for the bandaging. (Fig. 61, p. 114.) A folded pillow is placed under the thigh of the injured limb, so as to bend the knee and leave a deep space under the leg.

Bandaging the foot

1. The free end of the bandage is placed on the outer border of the foot with the front edge immediately behind the head of the 5th metatarsal bone. The bandage is passed inwards across the top of the foot with the front edge kept just behind the head of the 1st metatarsal bone. It is then carried under the foot and back to the starting point. Another complete turn of bandage is made in the same way.

2. The bandage is passed diagonally upwards and inwards over the top of the foot and front of the ankle to cover the inner side of the heel. It is then carried under the heel to the outer side.

3. The bandage is passed in a diagonal manner downwards and inwards to the inner border of the foot, so that it crosses the previous turn. It is then passed under the foot to the outer border.

4. The bandage is carried diagonally upwards and inwards across the front of the ankle, and passed round the inner side of the ankle and heel. It is then taken behind the ankle to the outer side. *See* Fig. 90.

Bandaging the leg

A series of simple spiral turns are taken round the leg until the upper border of the bandage reaches the tibial tubercle. Each turn of bandage covers the upper third of the previous turn, as shown in Fig. 90.

If possible, an additional turn is made over the final turn, so as to give the bandage a firm finish. The bandage is completed by being pinned off on the outer side of the leg. (Fig. 90.)

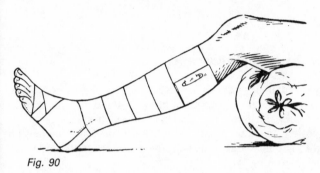

Fig. 90

Crêpe bandage support for foot and leg.

Sprain of the medial ligament

Sprains of the front and middle bands of fibres of the medial ligament of the ankle joint are treated in the same way as sprains of the lateral ligament. When support is used, however, and the ligament must be kept in a shortened position, the foot is held upwards and slightly inwards (dorsiflexion combined with slight inversion). To achieve an inversion pull on the foot, bandages and elastoplast strappings are started from the *inner* border, taken over the top of the foot, and then under the sole.

'Footballer's ankle'

Kicking a football often results in the front part of the capsule of the ankle joint being irritated by the constant stretching. This may cause increased bone-cell activity at the attachment of the capsule to the bone. Dorsiflexion of the ankle becomes limited and at times is painful. X-rays show an enlargement or 'lipping' of the bone on the front of the ankle.

In general, conservative treatment by physiotherapy is of little or no value. In some of the more severe cases operative treatment is necessary.

Chapter 9
Injuries of the knee ligaments

Injuries of the medial ligament

Sprains. The medial ligament is frequently sprained, either as the result of (*a*) an abduction strain, e.g. a blow on the outer side of the knee which forces the joint into the knock-knee position, or (*b*) a rotation strain, e.g. the knee is twisted while it is bent and the foot is taking weight. The ligament is usually injured close to its upper or femoral attachment. (Fig. 91.)

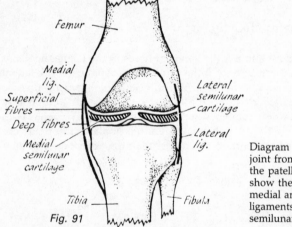

Diagram of the left knee joint from the front, with the patella removed, to show the position of the medial and lateral ligaments and the semilunar cartilages.

Fig. 91

For definition and degrees of sprain *see* p. 112.

Complete rupture. A complete tear of the medial ligament is uncommon. The usual cause of the tear is a violent abduction strain of the extended knee.

Involvement of semilunar cartilage. Severe injuries of the medial ligament are often complicated by tears of the medial semilunar cartilage, because the two structures are joined together.

1st degree or minor sprain

Main symptoms: Small amount of swelling; some pain on joint movement and slight loss of function.

Treatment: immediately after injury

The knee is supported by a crêpe bandage, which is applied in spica fashion, as described below. The player is allowed to walk, but must limit his activities for about 24 hours.

Crêpe bandage: divergent spica

A 3 in. crêpe bandage is applied to the knee in the form of a series of curves, or divergent spica turns, as shown in Fig. 96, p. 136. The bandage is arranged so that it is narrow at the back of the knee and broad at the sides and front.

Position of player. The spica may be applied with the player in lying or sitting, but the best position is half-lying on a massage couch (Fig. 61, p. 114). The thigh of the injured knee is supported by a folded pillow.

Tension of bandage. The bandage should be applied reasonably tightly, a firm degree of tension being exerted on each turn as it is carried round the knee. The turns behind the knee should be made to overlap each other as much as possible, so as to facilitate knee movements.

Bandaging technique

1. The end of the bandage is placed on the inner side of the knee, level with the patella. The bandage is then carried across the patella to the outer side of the joint. A piece of cotton wool, about 6 in. square, is placed behind the joint, and the bandage carried over it and round the joint to the starting point. Another turn of bandage is taken round the joint. (Fig. 92.)
2. The bandage is carried upwards and outwards in a curved direction, so that it covers the upper half of the previous turns. (Fig. 93.) The free end must be brought down level with the previous turns at the outer side of the joint, as demonstrated. The bandage is then passed behind the joint, over the previous turn, to the inner side of the knee.
3. The bandage is passed downwards and outwards in a curved direction, so that it covers the lower half of the straight turns. (Fig. 94.) It is then passed behind the joint to the inner side. It is important that the free end is brought down level with the straight turns at the outer side of the knee before it is passed behind the joint. Fig. 94 shows the

elliptical pattern which is formed on the front of the knee by the junction of the two curved turns.

4. The bandage is carried upwards and outwards, as described in para. 2, so that about three-quarters of the upper curved turn is covered. It is then taken behind the knee to the inner side.

5. The bandage is passed downwards and outwards, as described in para. 3, so that about three-quarters of the lower curved turn is covered. It is then passed behind the knee to the inner side.

6. The bandaging techniques described in paras. 4 and 5 are repeated. Fig. 95 shows the enlarged elliptical pattern on the front of the knee.

7. The remaining length of bandage is used up by taking one or two turns over the upper curved turn. The bandage is pinned off on the outer side of the knee, the free end being turned back on itself. (Fig. 96.) Any cotton wool projecting above or below the bandage at the back of the knee is pulled out.

Treatment: 24 hours after injury
(For period of about 7 days)

Physiotherapy. The crêpe bandage is removed and the medial ligament treated by heat therapy (preferably short-wave diathermy) and transverse frictions. Exercises are used to maintain the strength of the quadriceps muscle. Static exercises are used at first and progressed to dynamic movements.

Static exercises: (1) Contracting the quadriceps muscle of each thigh in turn from half-lying (Fig. 61, p. 114) or inclined long sitting (Fig. 97); each muscle group is contracted as strongly as possible, and slackened off fairly slowly. (2) As previous exercise, but as the quadriceps is contracted the ankle is bent strongly (dorsiflexion). (3) Each leg is raised in turn through 45° from half-lying or inclined long sitting; throughout the movement the knee must be kept firmly braced. (4) As previous exercise, but the movement of the injured limb is performed against a weight resistance.

Dynamic exercises: (1) Straightening each knee in turn from a sitting position on a massage couch or a table: full extension of the knee must be achieved. (2) As previous exercise, but the movement of the injured limb is performed against a weight resistance (Fig. 15, p. 49).

Support. The crêpe bandage is reapplied after treatment. It is discontinued after about two or three days.

Resuming training. When the player can use the knee normally the medial ligament is tested passively (p. 86); if the result is satisfactory, training is resumed. At each training session the knee should be supported by a divergent spica of elastoplast (Fig. 99); the same type

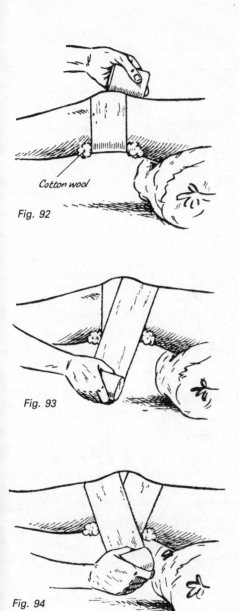

Fig. 92

Cotton wool

Fig. 93

Fig. 94

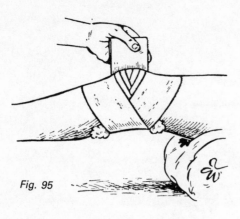

Fig. 95

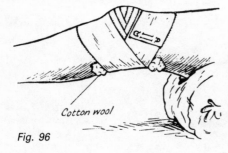

Cotton wool

Fig. 96

Figs. 92–96. Supporting the knee with a crêpe bandage: spica technique. The illustrations show the outer aspect of the left knee. Throughout the bandaging the heel rests on the massage couch or bed with the knee slightly flexed.

of strapping should be used when the player returns to the game. *See* p. 22.

Elastoplast strapping: divergent spica

The knee is strapped with 3 in. elastoplast, the same technique being used as described on p. 133, with the exception that the patella is not covered.

The strapping is started on the inner side of the joint, two elliptical turns being made, as shown in Fig. 98. To finish the strapping the elastoplast is cut on the inner side of the knee, and a small piece of zinc oxide strapping placed over it to prevent it from wrinkling up. Fig. 99 shows the completed strapping.

2nd degree or severe sprain

Main symptoms: Large amount of swelling; considerable pain and loss of function.

The injury should be seen by the club doctor as soon as possible.

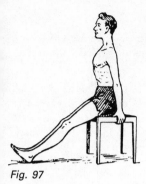

Fig. 97

Inclined long sitting: a useful starting position for static quadriceps exercises and straight leg raising movements.

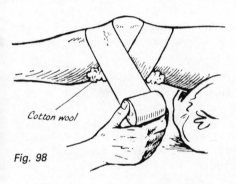

Cotton wool

Fig. 98

Outer aspect of left knee showing first two turns of elastoplast spica. The patella is left uncovered.

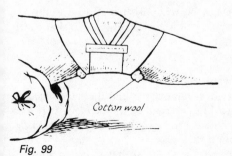

Cotton wool

Fig. 99

Inner aspect of left knee showing the completed spica strapping. A piece of zinc oxide adhesive plaster is stuck over the cut end of the elastoplast to prevent it from wrinkling up.

Treatment: immediately after injury

Strips of white lint soaked in lead lotion are placed round the knee joint. A pressure bandage is then applied, as described below. (Fig. 101, p. 140.)

Rest and elevation. The player should go to bed as soon as possible, and rest with the injured limb elevated on pillows. He must not take weight on the injured limb for at least 24 hours; when he has to walk he must use crutches. He should be instructed to loosen the bandage if the swelling increases and the bandage causes pain.

Pressure bandage

Four rectangular-shaped pieces of cotton wool are applied to the knee joint, each piece being compressed by horizontal turns of calico bandage. Each piece of wool is about 13 in. wide and of a length which enables it to be wrapped one and a half times round the knee: 26 in. is an approximate length. Two calico bandages are needed, 4 in. wide; the ends of the bandages are sewn together to make one long bandage. *See* p. 122.

Position of knee. The bandage is applied with the player in half-lying (Fig. 61, p. 114); a folded pillow is placed under the leg, to create a space under the knee, so that the bandaging can be carried out without the limb having to be constantly moved. The four pieces of cotton wool are placed on the thigh of the player's sound limb; the therapist can then reach them without having to release his grasp on the bandage.

Technique and precautions. The bandage is applied very tightly, the tension being increased as each piece of wool is added. When the bandage has been completed the circulation through the leg must be checked to see if it has been impaired in any way. *See* p. 123.

If varicose veins of the leg are present the veins must be drained and supported before the pressure bandage is applied. The limb is elevated on pillows for a few minutes, with the foot at a higher level than the hip. A crêpe bandage, 4 in. wide, is then applied to the leg from the webs of the toes to just below the knee joint, so that every part is covered (Fig. 90, p. 131).

Application of 1st piece of wool

1. The first piece of cotton wool is wrapped round the knee with the ends overlapping at the back. The free end of the bandage is placed on the inner side of the joint over the wool, *at the level of the patella.* Two turns are then taken round the knee.
2. The bandage is passed round the knee, so that it covers approxi-

mately the upper half of the previous turns and the adjoining area of cotton wool.

3. The bandage is taken round the knee again; it covers approximately the lower half of the original turns and the adjoining area of wool as shown in Fig. 100.

Application of 2nd piece of wool

1. The second piece of wool is added to the bandage. One end is placed at the back of the knee between the free end of the bandage and the previous turns. The remainder of the wool is then moulded round the knee, the loose end lying behind the free part of the bandage.

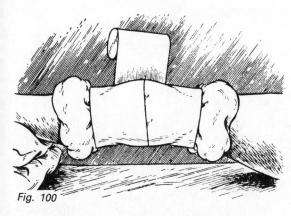

Pressure bandage for knee. The first layer of cotton wool has been covered. Note the wide free margins of wool.

Fig. 100

2. The bandage is carried round the knee, over the new wool; it encloses the loose end of the wool.

3. Two turns of bandage are taken round the joint as described in paras. 2 and 3 of the previous section.

Application of 3rd and 4th pieces of wool

The application of the wool and the bandaging technique are the same as described in the previous section.

Finishing the bandage

1. The lower edges of the four pieces of wool are turned back over the free edge of the bandage to a depth of about 3 in. If the wool is very bulky it may be thinned out with the fingers.

2. Two turns of bandage are taken round the knee, over the turn-over.

3. The upper edges of the wool layers are then turned over to a depth of about 2 in. Two turns of bandage are taken round the turn-over.

4. The remaining length of bandage is used to exert strong pressure over the wool padding. Spiral turns are made in a downward direction, each turn overlapping the previous one by two-thirds. When the lower border of the wool is reached the same process is repeated in an upward direction. The bandage is pinned off with a safety-pin on the outer side of the knee. (Fig. 101.)

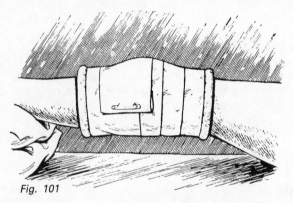

Fig. 101

The completed pressure bandage.

Treatment: 24 hours after injury

Physiotherapy. The bandage and lint strips are removed. Interferential therapy or short-wave diathermy is given with the injured limb elevated on pillows. Contrast bathing is also useful. The player must be encouraged to contract the quadriceps muscle statically in a 'little and often' manner throughout the day, and to carry out leg lifting exercises with the knee firmly braced. Quadriceps 'boosting' is of the greatest importance, because after any injury of the knee joint the muscle wastes rapidly and loses strength. Knee flexion exercises are not allowed because they tend to irritate the synovial membrane and increase the swelling.

Quadriceps inhibition. Sometimes after a knee injury it is impossible for the player to contract the quadriceps muscle or perform straight leg raising. This is because a contraction of the quadriceps would pull on the injured part and cause pain; the brain therefore automatically inhibits the action of the muscle.

Quadriceps inhibition must not be allowed to continue for long, because it increases the wasting of the muscle. The quadriceps should be stimulated by a surged faradic current, the strength used being sufficient to bring about a painless contraction. The player is instructed to 'attempt' to tighten up the quadriceps each time the muscle contracts in response to the current. If he does this conscientiously he will soon regain control of the muscle, and be able to exercise it normally. Faradism can then be discontinued.

Support. If the knee is badly swollen the pressure bandage should be reapplied, and the player advised to rest for a further 24 hours. If the swelling has subsided considerably the knee should be supported by a crêpe bandage: it is applied in spica fashion, as described on p. 133. The player is allowed to take weight on the injured limb, but should not stand or walk too much; at first he may have to use a stick. When sitting he should have the foot supported on a stool so that the leg is in a horizontal position.

Wedging of shoe worn on injured limb. The inner side of the heel is raised by about 3/16 in. or ¼ in. The raise is tapered off on the outer side, as shown in Fig. 102. When the player takes weight on the injured limb the wedge helps to close the inner side of the knee and prevents the medial ligament from being stretched.

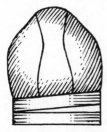

Method of wedging shoe heel so that the inner side is higher than the outer.

Fig. 102

Treatment: 48 hours after injury
(For a period of about 3 weeks)

Large effusion. If the joint is still very swollen interferential or heat therapy is used, together with static quadriceps exercises. The pressure bandage is reapplied after treatment, and the player is allowed to take weight on the injured limb, provided he does not overdo walking and standing. This regime is continued until the swelling has diminished.

Small or moderate effusion. If there is only a small or moderate degree of swelling present the medial ligament is treated by heat and transverse frictions. The quadriceps muscle is strengthened by static contractions and straight leg raising movements against weight resistance. Knee bending exercises are not allowed until the swelling has cleared up. Then the following types of exercises should be practised:

Strengthening exercises. (1) Knee stretching movements from sitting, with or without weight resistance (*see* p. 134), (2) heel raising and knee bending movements from standing, the arms being used at first to take some of the body-weight (Fig. 11, p. 47).

Mobility exercises. (1) Lying on massage couch, raising the thigh of the injured limb with heel in contact with the couch top, (2) lying face downwards on couch, bending each knee alternately, and (3) sitting over edge of massage couch or a table, bending and stretching the knees alternately. It is most important that all the exercises are performed within a pain-free range of movement.

Support. After treatment the knee is supported by a crêpe bandage, which is applied as a divergent spica (p. 133). Walking is allowed, the player being instructed to straighten the injured knee fully as he carries the leg forward.

Resuming training. At the end of about three weeks' treatment the medial ligament is tested passively (p. 86); if the test is satisfactory, training is resumed. At each training session the knee must be supported by an elastoplast strapping, as described on p. 136. The same type of strapping should be used when the player returns to the game. *See* p. 22.

Complete tear of medial ligament

Main symptoms: Rapid and large effusion of joint; considerable pain and almost complete loss of function; lateral instability of knee.

The injury must be seen by the club doctor as soon as possible.

Repair of ligament. When the ligament is ruptured it generally remains in its normal position; healing takes place if the knee is immobilized in a plaster cast for about 8 weeks. The cast extends from just above the ankle to the top of the thigh; the knee is fixed in almost full extension. Sometimes, however, the ligament is displaced downwards when it is ruptured, so that normal healing is impossible. Surgery is necessary; the torn end of the ligament is replaced and stitched in position. The knee is then immobilized for about 6 weeks in a plaster cast of the type previously described.

Treatment
1 When ligament is not displaced

When the cast is dry the player is allowed to take weight on the injured limb; he must be instructed to walk as normally as possible. It may be necessary for him to use a stick when he first starts to walk.

Exercise therapy. During the period in plaster the player must maintain the strength of the quadriceps muscle by practising all types of static quadriceps contractions and straight leg raising exercises. Static contractions should be performed on a 'little and often' basis.

'Attempted' knee stretching and bending movements are usually started after about a week. The player attempts to straighten the knee against the cast, 'holds' the quadriceps muscle in the contracted state for a moment, and then allows it to slacken off; he then attempts to bend the knee in the same manner. Exercises to maintain the strength of the hip and ankle muscles must also be practised.

Plaster cast removed. When the cast is removed, exercises are given to restore the mobility of the knee and increase the strength of the quadriceps and hamstring muscle group; the redevelopment of the quadriceps is especially important. Movements in water are extremely valuable, and the player should be encouraged to attend the swimming bath for leg exercises and swimming.

Heat and massage. Massage of the thigh and knee is used to disperse oedema (p. 130) and to assist in restoring knee movement. It should be preceded by 20 minutes' superficial heat therapy; hot packs are particularly useful. Transverse frictions are localized to the medial ligament in order to improve its mobility; scar tissue often tends to bind down the ligament to the underlying bone.

Preventing swelling. After the cast is removed the leg and knee should be supported by crêpe bandages for about 10 to 14 days. The leg bandage is applied from the webs of the toes to the tibial tubercle, as described on p. 130; the knee bandage is applied in spica fashion (p. 133). The player should remove the bandages at night when he goes to bed, and reapply them in the morning before he gets up.

Resuming training. About 4 to 6 weeks after the removal of the plaster cast the medial ligament is tested passively (p. 86); if the result is satisfactory, training is resumed. At each training session the knee must be strapped as described on p. 136; the same type of strapping should be used when the player returns to the game. *See* p. 22.

Treatment
2 When ligament is repaired by surgery

Treatment is much the same as described in the previous section, with the exception that the plaster cast is worn for 6 weeks and the player rests in bed for a few days after the operation. He is then allowed to bear weight on the injured limb, and is discharged from hospital. Static exercises to maintain the strength of the quadriceps muscle are started the day after the operation.

Traumatic ossification involving medial ligament

Sometimes when the upper attachment of the medial ligament of the knee is torn or bruised as the result of a blow, the underlying bone cells are aggravated and form a thin layer of new bone under the periosteum over the site of the injury. This new bone formation is known as Pellegrini-Stieda's disease.

When an injury of the medial ligament is not responding to treatment this condition should be suspected. It can only be detected by X-ray examination, however, and it is essential that the club doctor should be consulted about this as soon as possible. Meanwhile physiotherapy for the knee must be discontinued.

Treatment

The knee is immobilized for some weeks in a plaster cylinder which extends from just above the ankle to the groin. Normal walking is allowed, and static exercises to maintain the strength of the quadriceps are practised. Fixation of the knee is essential to enable the loose layer of bone to become firmly consolidated with the femur.

Injuries of the lateral ligament

Injuries of the lateral ligamen are less common than those of the medial ligament because (*a*) the ligament is relaxed when the knee is bent (which protects it from rotation strains), and (*b*) the knee is seldom forced into the adducted (bow-leg) position which puts the ligament on the stretch.

The ligament may be damaged at either point of attachment (Fig. 91, p. 132), but the lower is the commoner. Sometimes instead of the ligament being injured a fragment of the head of the fibula is torn away or avulsed.

Complete tears. When the lateral ligament is completely ruptured the knee joint is unstable and can be rocked sideways from the normal to the bow-leg position.

Treatment

Treatment is similar to that of injuries of the medial ligament (pp. 133–143). Wedging of the shoe is seldom necessary in the treatment of severe sprains (p. 141); if it is tried the outer side of the heel is built up.

Injuries of the cruciate ligaments

The cruciate ligaments (Fig. 40, p. 87) may be sprained or torn completely by a violent weight-bearing strain of the knee, e.g. the player turns sharply when he has all his weight on one foot which is fixed to the ground. They may also be injured by a stress which forces the knee joint into (a) hyperextension, or (b) abduction (knock-knee position). If the injury is due to an abduction strain the medial ligament is also injured.

The posterior or back cruciate ligament may also be stressed or torn completely by a violent blow over the front of the tibia which tends to drive it backwards into the popliteal space. The knee is generally in a flexed position when the injury occurs, because the ligament becomes taut on flexion of the knee.

It should be noted that a tear of the posterior cruciate ligament is much more disabling to the sportsman than one to the anterior or front cruciate ligament. This is because the forward thrust activity (as in sprinting) is impaired by the gross instability of the tibia on the femur.

For definition and degree of sprain *see* p. 112.

Sprain of front or back cruciate ligament

1st degree or minor sprain

Main symptoms: Small amount of swelling; some pain on knee movement, and slight loss of function.

Treatment: immediately after injury

The knee is supported by a crêpe bandage, which is applied in spica fashion as described on p. 133. The player is allowed to walk, but must limit his activities for 24 hours.

Treatment: 24 hours after injury
(For period of about 7 days)

Physiotherapy. The crêpe bandage is removed and the knee treated by short-wave diathermy. Exercises are used to maintain the strength of the quadriceps muscle, as described on p. 134. The crêpe bandage is reapplied after treatment; it is discontinued after about three days.

Resuming training. When the player can use the knee normally the injured ligament is tested passively (p. 86); training is resumed if the result is satisfactory. At each training session the knee should be supported by a divergent spica of elastoplast, as described on p. 136; the same type of support is used when the player returns to the game. *See* p. 22.

2nd degree or severe sprain

Main symptoms: Large amount of swelling; considerable pain and loss of function.

The club doctor should see the injury as soon as possible.

Treatment: immediately after injury

Strips of white lint soaked in lead lotion are placed round the knee joint; a pressure bandage is then applied as described on p. 138.

Rest and elevation. The player should go to bed as soon as possible and rest with the injured limb elevated on pillows. He must not take weight on the injured limb for at least 24 hours. *See* p. 138.

Treatment: 24 hours after injury

The pressure bandage is removed and either interferential therapy, standard or pulsed short-wave therapy is applied to the knee with the injured limb elevated. Static quadriceps contractions and straight leg raising exercises are used to maintain the strength of the quadriceps muscle, and are extremely important. *See* p. 134.

Quadriceps inhibition. If the player cannot contract the quadriceps normally, faradic stimulation is used as described on p. 140.

Support. If the knee is badly swollen the pressure bandage is reapplied, and the player advised to rest for a further 24 hours. If the swelling has subsided considerably the knee is supported by a crêpe bandage, as described on p. 133. Weight-bearing on the injured limb is allowed, but the player must not overdo standing or walking; he may have to use a stick at first.

Treatment: 48 hours after injury
(For period of about 5 to 6 weeks)

Large effusion. Short-wave diathermy is used, together with static quadriceps exercises. The pressure bandage is reapplied after treatment. The player is allowed to take weight on the injured limb, but is warned not to do too much standing or walking. This regime is continued until the swelling has subsided.

Small or moderate effusion. Short-wave diathermy is given, and the quadriceps muscle strengthened by static contractions and straight leg raising exercises against weight resistance. Knee flexion exercises are not allowed until the swelling has subsided. Then the movements described on p. 141 should be practised. All exercises must be kept within a pain-free range of movement.

Support. After treatment the knee is supported by a divergent spica bandage as described on p. 133. Walking is allowed; the player is instructed to extend the injured knee fully as he carries the leg forward.

Resuming training. At the end of 5 to 6 weeks' treatment the injured ligament is tested (p. 86); if the test is satisfactory (and the joint stable), training is resumed. At each training session the knee must be supported by an elastoplast strapping, as described on p. 136. The same type of strapping must be used when the player returns to the game. *See* p. 22.

Laxity of joint. The test may reveal some laxity of the knee. If the quadriceps is well developed and the joint cannot be moved passively in any direction when it is fully extended, training may be allowed. If the quadriceps is not strong enough to stabilize the knee, however, training must be postponed, and exercises for the thigh muscles – especially the quadriceps – intensified. Resisted exercises are essential.

Complete tear of front or back cruciate ligament

Main symptoms: Rapid and large effusion of knee; great pain and complete loss of function.

The injury must be seen by the club doctor as soon as possible.

Treatment

Complete rupture of a cruciate ligament is uncommon. The ligament will heal satisfactorily if it is protected by immediate and complete immobilization. The knee is fixed (in slight flexion) in a plaster cast which extends from the webs of the toes to just below the groin. The cast is worn for about 3 months.

The healed ligament rarely regains its previous strength and tautness, and this gives rise to some degree of instability of the knee. Instability can be controlled by developing the thigh muscles, particularly the quadriceps.

In neglected tears, and when the injury has failed to heal in spite of treatment by immobilization, the knee joint may be so unstable that sport will be impossible. Operations designed to replace the torn ligament have been tried, but are seldom completely satisfactory. A new ligament is constructed from the fascia lata of the thigh: a strip of fascia (still attached to its lower end) is passed through drill holes in the femur and tibia in such a way that it crosses the knee in the position normally occupied by the ligament. Unfortunately, a fascial 'ligament' tends to stretch and the knee becomes unstable.

Exercise therapy during period of immobilization. As for torn medial ligament, p. 142.

Physiotherapy when plaster cast is removed. As for torn medial ligament (p. 143), but transverse frictions are not used.

Chapter 10
Other injuries of the knee

Traumatic synovitis of the knee

Traumatic synovitis or 'water on the knee' consists of an inflammation of the synovial membrane of the joint (Fig. 41, p. 87), which results in the formation of an excessive amount of synovial fluid. The distension of the synovial pouch obliterates the normal joint hollows, and the patella can be made to 'tap' against the underlying femoral condyles. The knee swells gradually over a period of several hours.

Synovitis can occur as a separate condition – the result, for example, of a kick on the knee – or in association with other knee injuries, e.g. sprain of a ligament or nipping of one of the semilunar cartilages.

Treatment

The treatment of traumatic synovitis is summarized here, because in many ways it resembles the treatment of sprains of the knee (p. 133). Progress, however, is far more rapid.

When the swelling is developing. A pressure bandage is applied to the knee, as described on p. 138, to restrict the formation of synovial fluid, and the player is warned not to bend or stretch the knee because movement irritates the synovial membrane. When the knee is badly swollen the player should rest in bed or on a couch for 24 to 48 hours with the injured limb elevated on pillows. When the swelling is less severe he should do as little walking and standing as possible, and remember to keep the knee stiff. In sitting he should 'keep the leg up' by supporting it on a broad stool or chair.

Resting the limb in an elevated position helps to disperse the synovial effusion by aiding the circulation through the veins and lymphatics of the thigh. This is important, because the swelling disorganizes the lymphatic drainage system of the knee, which normally removes any excess synovial fluid.

Static quadriceps exercises. Static contractions of the quadriceps are practised 'little and often' with the limb elevated; straight leg raising should also be carried out with the knee firmly braced (p. 134). The exercises not only help to maintain the strength of the quadriceps muscle but assist the returning circulation through the thigh; the alternate contraction and relaxation of the quadriceps acts as a kind of automassage on the veins and lymphatic vessels.

Dynamic quadriceps exercises in which the knee is bent and stretched are taboo, for the reason previously given.

When the swelling has subsided, or almost subsided. The pressure bandage is discarded, and the knee supported by a crêpe bandage as described on p. 133. The bandage is worn for a few days only to accustom the knee to being without support.

Normal knee movements are allowed, but the player should be warned not to overtax the joint at first; in particular he should not do too much walking. Strengthening exercises for the quadriceps are essential; straight leg raising is performed against weight resistance, and dynamic exercises are introduced, e.g. knee stretching from sitting, with or without weight resistance, and heel raising and knee bending movements from standing, the arms being used at first to take some of the body-weight (Fig. 11, p. 47). The dynamic exercises must be progressed very carefully; they should be discontinued at once if there is any increase or return of effusion. Static exercises are then used until the swelling subsides.

Mobility exercises. Exercises to restore knee flexion are seldom needed. When the effusion has been severe, however, and knee movements have been restricted for several days, flexion exercises may be helpful. *See* Figs. 20–23, p. 57.

Resuming training. Training is resumed when the quadriceps has regained its normal strength and efficiency. The knee does not need to be strapped for training or play.

Haemarthrosis of the knee
(Bleeding into the joint)

A severe blow on the knee may tear the blood vessels of the synovial membrane, and cause bleeding into the joint. Haemarthrosis also accompanies fractures of the patella and tibial spine.

In haemarthrosis swelling is rapid and may occur within an hour. The swelling is firmer than in synovitis, pain is greater and the joint feels hot; the temperature of the body rises to between 38° and 39°C (100° and 102°F).

Haemarthrosis is a serious condition. The player should be seen by the club doctor as soon as possible; if he is not available the player should be sent to the nearest hospital.

Chondromalacia patellae

The cartilage on the articular side of the patella becomes roughened; on examination a grating sound is heard during movement of the knee joint.

The patient will complain although the knee joint is normal. The pain is more marked when walking up and down stairs and walking down slopes, and is severe when the patella is pressed down on the femur or moved from side to side. The lesion often progresses to osteoarthritis. Diagnosis is confirmed by X-ray examination.

Chondromalacia patellae is fairly common in individuals who engage in body-contact sports; it is possibly due to a direct blow or repeated minor injuries involving the patella. The condition also occurs in young athletes who have a tendency to knock-knee and genu recurvatum (hyperextension of the knee). A previous injury affecting the knee can also lead to the condition if rehabilitation has been inadequate and led to a marked weakness of the quadriceps muscle.

Mechanical factor. It should be noted that weakness of the vastus medialis muscle causes an altered alignment of pull on the patella, causing it to be shifted slightly laterally when the knee is extended by the action of vastus lateralis and the tensor fascia latae muscles.

Treatment

The condition is alleviated to some extent by a period of rest from high-level activity, combined with short-wave therapy and exercise therapy directed at strengthening the vastus medialis. Exercises are also used to maintain the mobility of the knee.

It is essential that quadriceps exercises, both free and resisted, should take place through the last 30° of knee extension. During each movement great emphasis must be laid on securing the final degrees of extension to ensure that the vastus medialis is totally activated.

Surgery. Surgical intervention is sometimes necessary. Procedures used are: (a) the affected articular cartilage of the patella is smoothed off; (b) the lateral aspect of the patella is released (lateral release); and (c) in severe cases it may be necessary to remove the patella.

Chapter 11

Tears of the semilunar cartilages

The semilunar cartilages are two fibro-cartilages which lie between the head of the tibia and the condyles of the femur, as shown in Fig. 40, p. 87. They assist in the lubrication of the knee and act as shock absorbers; they also deepen the surface of the tibia for the condyles of the femur, and facilitate twisting movements of the joint.

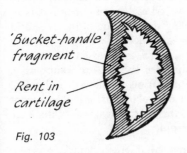

'Bucket-handle' fragment

Rent in cartilage

Fig. 103

'Bucket-handle' tear of semilunar cartilage: the 'bucket-handle' fragment is displaced towards the centre of the knee joint.

Mechanics of injury

Injuries of the semilunar cartilages are caused by the knee being rotated strongly while it is partly flexed and carrying the body-weight. The twist of the femur on the tibia exerts a grinding, compression force which tears or splits the cartilage. The tear may extend along the whole length of the cartilage (Fig. 103) or be confined to the front or back part. The medial cartilage is torn much more often than the lateral.

Sometimes a fragment of the torn cartilage is displaced towards the middle of the joint; the knee then 'locks' in the semiflexed position, because the torn portion of the cartilage is nipped by the femur and the tibia during extension. When the tear is confined to the back part of the cartilage, or to the central free edge, 'locking' seldom occurs.

Main symptoms of torn cartilage

When 'locking' occurs. The knee swells rapidly and the distension of the joint may become extreme if the displaced cartilage is left unreduced for long. Attempted extension of the joint produces pain.

The player should be seen at once by the club doctor; if this is not possible he should be sent to hospital. It is essential that a medical man should see the player with the knee 'locked', so that a diagnosis of torn cartilage may be established. If the trainer manipulates the knee and reduces the displaced cartilage valuable clinical evidence is lost.

When 'locking' does not occur. There may be a small or large amount of swelling. The player complains that the knee feels unstable; pain is referred to the inner or outer aspects of the joint, depending on whether the medial or lateral cartilage is involved.

The player should be seen as soon as possible by the club doctor.

Treatment

Torn cartilage with 'locking'. The club doctor or the casualty officer of the local hospital reduces the displaced cartilage by manipulation. Treatment is then directed at dispersing the swelling of the knee and maintaining the strength of the quadriceps muscle. Pressure bandaging, rest and static quadriceps exercises are used for the first 24 to 48 hours. As the swelling subsides the pressure support is replaced by a crêpe bandage, weight-bearing is allowed and active movements of the knee are started. In general, the pattern of treatment follows that described for a sprain of the medial ligament of the knee (pp. 138–142), but progress is more rapid.

Operation. If the cartilage is not removed (meniscectomy) recurrent displacement occurs and the player feels that at any time the knee may 'let him down'. Repeated displacement of the cartilage scars the joint surfaces and leads to early osteoarthritis.

Two types of operative procedures may be followed. In one the torn cartilage is removed in its entirety. In the other, an arthroscopic examination of the knee is carried out and the torn portion of the cartilage removed. Today, this procedure is used more frequently than the removal of the entire cartilage.

Rehabilitation will depend on the type of surgery used (pp. 153 and 154).

It should be noted that peripheral tears of the cartilages can be repaired successfully by suturing. A good result can be expected, because the peripheral portion of the cartilage has a blood supply. The lesion will therefore heal satisfactorily.

Suspected tear of cartilage without 'locking'. Treatment is given to disperse the swelling and maintain the strength of the quadriceps, as previously outlined. When the joint has returned to normal the club doctor usually suggests that the player should resume training and 'try out' the knee by performing all types of vigorous activities which throw a rotation strain on the joint, e.g. running (stopping suddenly with a turn to one side), quick full squats, and jumping over a succession of low objects, such as forms.

During this 'provocative' training the injured cartilage may be displaced again, and this is usually accepted as evidence that the cartilage is torn and should be removed. If displacement does not occur the player is allowed to return to the game. It is more than probable that if the cartilage is torn it will be displaced at some time during play; failing this, reactionary swelling and pain will occur after the game.

Treatment after operation

1. Complete removal of cartilage. Orthopaedic surgeons differ with regard to the type of immobilization and management employed in the post-operative phase of treatment. Three main regimes are widely used: (a) Non-weight-bearing regime, (b) Early weight-bearing regime (after 5 days), and (c) Early weight-bearing regime (with plaster cylinder or wrap-around back splint).

Only the *non-weight-bearing regime* is described here.

First 10 days. The surgeon removes the torn cartilage through a small incision, about ½ to 2 in. in length. Immediately after the operation he applies a firm pressure bandage to the knee, and this is worn until the stitches are removed in about 10 days' time. The bandage maintains the knee in extension and prevents bleeding into the joint.

Early exercise treatment. The patient rests in bed for about two or three days until he has good quadriceps control and can perform straight leg raising satisfactorily. During this time he will be encouraged to carry out all types of static exercises. In some hospitals weight-resisted straight leg raising exercises are started about two days after the operation.

After about the third post-operative day the patient is allowed out of bed for short periods of walking and sitting. When sitting the affected limb must be supported in a horizontal position by a stool and pillows. Walking is restricted to a non-weight-bearing technique with elbow crutches.

Non-weight-bearing is continued until the stitches are removed on about the tenth post-operative day. During this phase the patient may be discharged home or remain in the ward.

Progression. After the stitches have been removed a crêpe bandage is applied to the knee joint to control oedema and provide some degree of support. The patient then makes a gradual progression from partial to full weight-bearing. He is warned not to walk or stand too much for the first few days or the knee may swell badly.

The crêpe bandage is applied in spica (p. 133) or figure-of-eight fashion. It is generally worn for about 7 to 10 days.

Intensive exercise therapy is then required for about 4 weeks to build up the strength of the quadriceps and restore the mobility of the knee; the muscles of the hip and ankle must also be developed. The player either attends the hospital physiotherapy department or is treated by the club therapist or trainer.

Knee flexion exercises. Knee bending exercises must not be given too soon or they may cause recurrent swelling and delay recovery. In general, they may be started about 10 days after the player is discharged from hospital; if the knee is swollen, however, they must be postponed. Some non-weight-bearing exercises are illustrated in Figs. 20 to 22, p. 57. A useful weight-bearing exercise to restore the final degrees of knee flexion is shown in Fig. 23, p. 57.

In restoring knee movements after meniscectomy it is important to remember that knee flexion will return gradually without any difficulty. Forced movements and exercises which cause pain must never be given.

Quadriceps exercises. Strengthening exercises for the quadriceps must be restricted to static contractions (p. 134) and straight leg raising against weight resistance until knee movements are allowed. Dynamic quadriceps exercises are then introduced and progressed smoothly from non-weight-bearing (p. 134) to resisted movements (Fig. 15, p. 49) and full weight-bearing movements, e.g. heel raising and knee bending.

Resuming training. At the end of a month's treatment (provided the knee is free from swelling and the quadriceps is well developed) training is resumed. At each training session the knee must be supported by an elastoplast strapping, as described on p. 136. The same type of strapping should be used when the player returns to the game in about two weeks' time. *See* p. 22.

Note. From time to time other injuries involving the knee joint occur in association with a cartilage lesion, e.g. sprain of a cruciate ligament or of the medial ligament. These injuries can lead to some instability of the joint, and in consequence the rehabilitation programme will have to be extended. In some instances the laxity of the joint can lead to an abrupt termination of the player's career.

2. Partial removal of cartilage by arthroscopy. The achievement of full function is much more rapid than after a complete removal of the cartilage. For example, the patient is capable of walking freely two or three days after the operation. He will have good control of the knee joint and there will be very little effusion. The rehabilitation programme can therefore proceed at a more rapid pace.

Reassuring the player

With good surgery, and adequate after-treatment by exercises, the player who has had a torn cartilage either partially or completely removed will find that his knee will be as sound as before the injury, and perfectly capable of being used for all types of vigorous sport, including first-class football. It is most important.that he should be reassured about this, because he is often extremely apprehensive about the future efficiency of the joint.

Chapter 12

Injuries of the thigh and leg muscles

Muscle and tendon injuries may be divided into two main groups: (1) Minor injuries which can be treated successfully by physiotherapy and support, such as strains, tearing of some of the muscle or tendon fibres, and muscle bruising; and (2) Severe injuries, such as complete muscle tears, which require surgical treatment.

Minor injuries

Muscle and tendon strains. Muscle and tendon strains are caused by over-use or excessive stretching, and give rise to stiffness and pain. Contrary to the generally accepted view the injured structures are not torn; the symptoms are due to protective muscle spasm and a mild localized inflammation.

Teno-synovitis and tendinitis. Strains of tendons may give rise to teno-synovitis or tendinitis. The tendons around the ankle are often affected, e.g. teno-synovitis of the tendons of the tibialis anterior and peronei muscles, and tendinitis of the Achilles tendon. (Figs. 37 and 38, p. 84.) 'Creaking' or crepitus can often be detected.

Tearing of some of the muscle fibres. Tears of the quadriceps, hamstrings, adductors and calf muscles are common. The fibres are torn as the result of (*a*) momentary incoordination of the muscle (which is particularly likely to occur when the athlete or player is tiring), or (*b*) arrested contraction of the muscle by some outside force, e.g. a player about to kick a ball gets his foot 'trapped' by another player, and the action of the quadriceps is halted abruptly. The main belly of the muscle may be torn or the area where it joins with its tendon; the injury is often associated with a tearing of some of the fibres of the overlying fascia. The main symptoms consist of localized swelling, pain and some loss of function.

Formation of haematoma. Muscle tears are always associated with a rupturing of some of the small blood vessels of the damaged area, which leads to the formation of a collection of blood in the muscle, known as a haematoma. The clotting of the blood after a short time checks the bleeding from the torn blood vessels, and links together the ends of the torn muscle fibres, thus preparing the way for repair by fibrous scar tissue (p. 16). The escaped blood seeps between the tissue layers and often spreads for a considerable distance. This explains the frequent appearance of bruising in places some distance from the damaged area, e.g. above the knee when the injury is to the middle of the quadriceps or hamstrings.

Muscle bruising or haematoma. This is a very common injury in soccer, rugby and boxing. It is generally caused by a direct blow, but it can also be the result of a fall on hard ground. The small blood vessels of the damaged area of the muscle are torn, so that a blood clot or haematoma forms in the muscle, as described above. The symptoms are similar to those of a muscle tear – pain, localized swelling and some loss of function. In soccer and rugby the quadriceps muscle is involved more frequently than any of the other muscle groups.

Traumatic ossification. In severe bruising of the quadriceps the periosteal covering of the femur may be damaged, resulting in increased bone-cell activity. A detached plaque of new bone is formed, and if the injured part is not rested further ossification occurs. The resulting bony mass interferes severely with the function of the quadriceps muscle and knee joint.

Muscle and tendon strains

Treatment

Muscle strains usually clear up without any treatment. If treatment is necessary it follows the lines recommended for tearing of some of the fibres; recovery is far more rapid.

Teno-synovitis and tendinitis. Doctors differ as to what is the best type of treatment for these conditions. Some advocate complete rest of the tendon (by plaster fixation of the joint on which the tendon acts); others recommend short-wave diathermy and transverse frictions. Treatment by deep friction is painful but often extremely effective; when the massage is given it is most important that the tendon should be kept on the stretch.

Tendonitis of Achilles tendon. When a tendinitis of the Achilles tendon is treated by heat and transverse frictions the tendon should be relieved of as much strain as possible when the player is standing and walking.

To do this the shoe heel should be raised temporarily by about $3/16$ in.; alternatively a thick piece of felt or sponge-rubber can be worn inside the shoe under the heel.

Mid-thigh tear of some of the fibres of the hamstrings or quadriceps

Treatment: immediately after injury

The thigh is supported by a pressure bandage, which is applied in spiral fashion, as described below. Crêpe bandages are often used to give pressure instead of the calico bandages recommended for ligamentous sprains.

Rest and elevation. If the tearing appears to be fairly extensive the player should go to bed as soon as possible and rest for about 24 hours with the limb elevated on pillows; if, on the other hand, the tear is of a comparatively minor nature the player is allowed to walk but must limit his activities for at least 24 hours. He must be instructed to loosen the pressure bandage if the swelling increases and the bandage causes pain.

Pressure bandage

Four rectangular-shaped pieces of cotton wool are applied to the thigh, each piece being compressed by spiral turns of crêpe bandage. Each piece of wool is about 13 in. wide and of a length which enables it to be wrapped one and a half times round the thigh; 30 in. is an approximate length. Two crêpe bandages are needed, 4 in. wide.

Position of thigh. The bandage is applied with the player in half-lying (Fig. 61, p. 114); a folded pillow is placed under the leg, to create a space under the thigh, so that the bandaging can be done without the limb having to be moved constantly. The four pieces of wool are placed on the thigh of the player's sound limb; the therapist can then reach them without having to release his grasp on the bandage.

Technique and precautions. The bandage is applied very tightly, the tension being increased as each piece of wool is applied. When the bandage has been completed the circulation of the part must be checked to see if it has been impaired in any way (p. 123). If varicose veins of the leg are present the veins must be drained and supported before the pressure bandage is applied, as described on p. 138.

Application of 1st piece of wool
1. The first piece of wool is wrapped round the thigh with the ends

overlapping on the inner side. The upper border of the wool should reach to about the crutch, and the lower border well below the knee.

2. The end of the bandage is placed below the knee, on its inner aspect, with the lower edge about an inch above the lower border of the wool. Two or three turns of bandage are taken round the knee and lower thigh.

3. Simple spiral turns of bandage are then taken up the thigh, each turn covering about two-thirds of the previous turn. The upper limit of the bandage should be about 1½ in. from the crutch; this leaves a margin of wool uncovered.

Application of 2nd piece of wool

1. The second piece of wool is added to the bandage. One end is placed on the inner side of the thigh between the free end of the bandage and the previous turns. The remainder of the wool is then moulded round the thigh, the loose end lying behind the free end of the bandage.

2. A turn of bandage is made round the thigh over the wool; it encloses the loose end of the wool.

3. Simple spiral turns of bandage are made down the thigh, each turn overlapping the previous turn by about two-thirds. The final turn should be made at the same level as the original starting turn.

Application of 3rd and 4th pieces of wool

The application of the wool and the bandaging technique are the same as described in the previous section.

Finishing the bandage

1. The lower edges of the four pieces of wool are turned over the bandage; if they are very bulky they can be thinned out with the fingers. Two turns of bandage are taken round the thigh, over the turn-over of wool; this makes a firm, neat border.

2. Spiral turns of bandage are then taken up the thigh to the upper limit of the bandage. The upper edges of the four layers of cotton wool are turned over the bandage in the same manner as the lower edges. Two turns of bandage are taken round the thigh, over the turn-over.

3. If there is only a small amount of bandage left the end is pinned off just below the turn-over. If a fair amount of bandage is left over it is used up by spiral turns being taken round the thigh in a downward direction. The end is pinned off on the outer side of the thigh.

Treatment: 24 hours after injury

Physiotherapy. The pressure bandage is removed and the injured area treated by either pulsed or standard short-wave therapy, ultrasound or interferential therapy. When electrotherapy apparatus of this type is not available contrast bathing is a very useful treatment.

The thigh is then massaged in a general manner, kneading and effleurage being used only. If the tear has been severe it is best to avoid the injured area for a day or so; otherwise the massage manipulations should gradually encroach on it.

The player is treated in the prone or face-downwards position if the hamstrings have been torn, and in half-lying (Fig. 61, p. 114) if the quadriceps muscle has been injured. In the prone position the legs are supported by a pillow, so that the knees are flexed to about 45°; this relaxes the hamstrings.

Static contractions of the injured muscle are practised. To contract the hamstrings with ease the muscles must first be placed in a shortened position, e.g. the prone position suggested above or half-lying with the knees bent to about 45°; the player then attempts to bend each knee in turn without actually moving the joint. Static quadriceps exercises are described on p. 134.

Muscle inhibition. After a severe tear the player may find it difficult or impossible to contract the injured muscle because of reflex inhibition (p. 140). The muscle should then be stimulated by a surged faradic current, the strength being sufficient to bring about a painless contraction. Faradism is discontinued when the player regains control of the muscle.

Support. At the end of the treatment session the thigh is supported by a reinforced elastoplast strapping, as described on p. 162. Strapping is used until the muscles are capable of normal activity without support.

The player is allowed to take weight on the injured limb, but at first should not stand or walk too much. This is particularly important if the injury has been severe.

Progressing treatment. As the acuteness of the injury subsides the massage is deepened and the injured area treated by transverse and circular frictions. Exercises are given to strengthen the injured muscle and maintain the mobility of the knee; they must be progressed smoothly from free, non-weight-bearing movements to resisted and weight-bearing exercises. Until the torn fibres are healed (in approximately 10 days from the time of injury) the movements must be kept within a pain-free range, and the muscle must not be stretched in any way. After this time, however, exercises should be introduced which *gradually* put the muscle on the stretch, so that it regains its normal power of extensibility. Unless this is done the player may well suffer a recurrence of the injury when he resumes training.

Strengthening exercises. A series of progressive exercises for the hamstrings is given here; quadriceps exercises are described on pp. 134 and 141. The majority of these exercises maintain knee movement.

Hamstring exercises. (1) Bending each knee in turn through 45° to 90° from the prone or face-downwards position; (2) Raising each leg in turn a short distance backwards from the prone position with the knee *kept straight*; (3) Bending the knee of the injured limb while standing on the sound leg with the hands grasping a chair back or a wall-bar: the movement is taken as far as possible without producing pain; (4) As previous exercise, but when the knee is bent to 90° the thigh is raised backwards with the knee 'held' in position; (5) As Ex. 4, but performed from prone lying; (6) As Ex. 1, but a weight-shoe is worn on the foot of the injured limb; the knee is bent to a right angle.

Restoring muscle extensibility when repair has taken place

Hamstrings. The hamstrings are stretched gently when, from lying, the player raises the leg through 45° with the knee kept straight; further stretching is achieved by raising the leg still higher, provided the therapist holds the pelvis and prevents it from tilting backwards.

More advanced extensibility techniques are as follows: (1) In standing, with one foot a pace in front of the other, the player bends slowly forwards and attempts to touch the front of the leading foot. When stretching the left hamstring muscles the left foot is placed in the forward position; in stretching the right hamstring muscles the right foot occupies the forward position. (2) The player sits on a massage couch with one leg over the side (foot resting on the floor) and the other leg resting straight along the length of the couch. He reaches forwards to touch the toes of this leg. Thus, to stretch the right hamstring muscles the right leg rests on the couch, and *vice versa*.

Quadriceps. A gentle stretching for the quadriceps muscle as a whole consists of the player bending the knee through about 90° from prone lying; further stretching is achieved by increasing the range of knee flexion. More advanced extensibility exercises are carried out in kneeling and kneel-sitting: (1) From kneeling the player lowers the trunk backwards to sit on the heels; (2) From the kneel-sitting position (sitting on the heels) the player lowers his trunk slowly backwards towards the floor, supporting his hands on the floor if necessary, so as to assume an arch position. This is a particularly useful exercise to employ when it is necessary to stretch the rectus femoris (commonly involved in thigh injuries). It brings about extension of the hip and flexion of the knee: two movements which place the rectus femoris fibres under stress.

Resuming training. After about 6 weeks' treatment following a severe tear the injured muscle is tested against manual resistance, as described on p. 88; it is also tested to see if full extensibility has been regained;

if the results are satisfactory, training is resumed.

For minor tears the same procedure is carried out after about 2 to 3 weeks' treatment.

At each training session the injured muscle must be supported either by a reinforced elastoplast strapping, as described below, or a zinc oxide strapping (p. 163). The same type of strapping must be used when the player returns to the game. *See* p. 22.

Limitation of strapping. It is important to realize that the strappings do not keep the injured muscle in a relaxed, protected position, but merely support it in a circular fashion, as shown in Figs. 104 and 106. When full movement of the knee is required it is impossible to strap the thigh muscles so that they cannot be put on the stretch.

Reinforced elastoplast strapping

Elastoplast strapping. The thigh is strapped with 3 in. elastoplast, the strapping extending well above and below the injured area, so that the thigh is not constricted in any way. A simple spiral technique is used, each turn overlapping the previous one by about a third of its width. (Fig. 104.) The elastoplast should be applied reasonably tightly, a firm degree of tension being exerted on each turn as it is taken round the thigh.

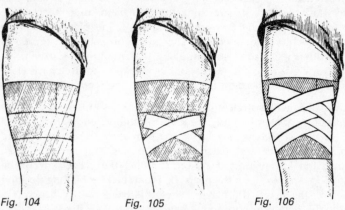

Fig. 104   Fig. 105   Fig. 106

Fig. 104. Elastoplast strapping for the quadriceps or hamstrings.

Fig. 105. Reinforcing the elastoplast support: the first strap of zinc oxide plaster in position.

Fig. 106. The completed reinforced strapping.

The strapping is best applied with the player in half-lying (Fig. 61, p. 114). A folded pillow is placed under the leg, so as to leave a deep space under the thigh.

Zinc oxide strapping. Three strips of 2 in. zinc oxide adhesive plaster are moulded over the elastoplast strapping, as shown in Fig. 106. The strips should be long enough to encircle the thigh with the ends crossing on the front, as illustrated; an approximate length is 27 in. The easiest method of assessing a basic length for the strips is to use a tape measure round the thickest part of the thigh.

To achieve a good strapping the therapist must allow the straps to more or less follow the contours of the muscles in their own way once he has positioned them behind the thigh. The strap ends are moulded *separately* round the thigh, and the therapist must not put tension on both ends at once. The straps should lie flush with the elastoplast covering; 'wrinkles' are not allowed.

Application of 1st strap. The first strap is applied behind the thigh well below the injured area. The inner end is taken across the front of the thigh in a slanting direction; the outer end is then carried across it. Fig. 105, p. 162.

Application of 2nd and 3rd straps. The second and third straps are applied in the same manner as the first strap, but each strap overlaps the previous one by about a third of its width. Fig. 106, p. 162.

Zinc oxide strapping

Four strips of 2 in. zinc oxide adhesive plaster are moulded round the thigh so that they cover the injured area and extend well above and below it. *See* Fig. 106. In this way the strapping acts as a broad, supporting band, and not as a narrow constricting belt. For technique of application *see* previous zinc oxide strapping.

Mid-thigh tear of some of the fibres of the hip adductor muscles

Mid-thigh tears of the hip adductors (Fig. 44, p. 90) are treated in the same manner as tears of the hamstrings and quadriceps (pp. 158–163). In applying the reinforced elastoplast or zinc oxide strapping (pp. 162–163) an attempt should be made to give special support to the inner side of the thigh. To do this each zinc oxide strap is positioned so that there is a greater length of strapping on the inner side of the thigh than on the outer, and the two ends cross on the outer side of the thigh. In general only three strips of zinc oxide strapping are required.

Limitation of strappings. Because of the importance of allowing hip movement the adductor muscles can only be supported in a circular fashion; any attempt to strap them in a shortened position would necessitate limiting hip movement.

Exercise therapy. Some examples of progressive exercises to strengthen the adductor mucles are given here: (1) Pressing the knees together from lying or half-lying; (2) Parting the thighs from crook lying (knees bent to about 90°), closing them and pressing the knees together strongly; (3) Crossing the injured leg over the front of the sound leg while standing in front of a chair back or wall-bar (the hands grasp the chair back or wall-bar); and (4) As previous exercise, but the injured leg is raised sideways as far as possible before it is carried in front of the sound leg.

Restoring muscle extensibility. When repair has taken place the following exercises should be practised: (1) Lying on the floor or a massage couch, parting *both* legs as much as possible; (2) Standing with legs well astride, bending the trunk slowly forwards and downwards to touch the floor through the legs; and (3) Stretching of left or right adductor groups. *Left adductors*: from a wide-stride standing position the player allows the right knee to bend sideways, while he keeps the right foot on the floor and the left knee straight. *Right adductors*: same exercise, but the left knee is bent slowly.

Strains of musculo-tendinous origin of hip adductors

The results of treatment are often extremely poor, sometimes because the origin of the adductor muscles is allowed to shorten to a considerable extent.

Note. When the symptoms of adductor strain persist, attention should be given to the symphysis pubis joint. Instability of this joint gives rise to similar symptoms to that of adductor strain, and the two are often confused.

Specific X-ray examination is essential to ascertain the stability of the symphysis joint. The X-ray should be taken with the patient standing on one leg on a raised platform, so that any joint instability which exists will be clearly demonstrated.

On occasions pain in the region of the symphysis pubis can be caused by low-grade infection of the area, or even by a stress hernia. *See* p. 80.

Treatment

A strain of the tendinous origin of the hip adductors is treated in much the same way as tears of the hamstrings and quadriceps (pp. 158–163), but there are certain important differences.

Immediately after injury. Complete rest or very limited activity is advised for 24 hours, depending on the severity of the injury. No attempt is made to support the injured tendon (*see* Support, below).

24 hours after injury. Pulsed short-wave therapy is localized to the injured tendon in the groin. Transverse frictions are then applied to the tendon with the hips fully abducted – the player lies on his back on the massage couch, with the thighs fully astride and the knees bent so that the lower legs hang over the sides of the couch. Active treatment is started to maintain the extensibility of the adductor muscles as a whole. At first, leg parting movements are practised in water, the player using the club bath or a swimming pool. It is essential that he is instructed to part both legs, and is warned not to concentrate on moving the injured limb only.

Progression. Pulsed short-wave therapy and transverse frictions are given daily. As the acuteness of the injury subsides the player practises the exercises and activities described on p. 164 for increasing the extensibility of the hip adductors.

Support. There is no sound method of supporting the injury by strapping. This is solely because of the position of the adductor tendons in the groin.

Resuming training. With good treatment the player will generally be able to resume training after about 5 weeks. Before training is started the hip adductors are tested, as described on p. 91.

Tears of some of the fibres of the belly of the calf muscles

Tears of some of the fibres of the belly of the calf muscles are treated in the same manner as tears of the hamstrings and quadriceps (pp. 158–163), with the exception that a crêpe bandage is used instead of a pressure support. The bandage is applied from the webs of the toes to just below the knee, as described on p. 130. A heel lift (p. 158) is used to relieve the calf muscles of strain when the player is standing or walking.

Strapping. About 24 hours after injury the crêpe bandage is replaced by a zinc oxide strapping of the type described on p. 166, or a reinforced elastoplast strapping. The same type of support is used when training and play are resumed. *See* p. 22.

Physiotherapy. When the calf muscles are treated by heat and massage

the player takes up the prone or face-downwards position, with the
leg supported by a folded pillow so that the knee is flexed to about
45°. Strengthening exercises for the calf muscles are described on p. 46.

Restoring muscle extensibility when repair has taken place. (1) To
stretch both calf muscles the player stands facing a wall and about a
yard away from it. He leans forwards from the ankles to place the
palms of his hands flat on the wall, and then carries out a number of
slow arm bending and stretching movements. During the arm movements it is essential that the heels are not to be raised from the floor;
the knees must also be kept straight. (2) To stretch the left or right calf
muscles the player stands with one foot a pace in front of the other,
toes pointing forwards, and slowly bends the forward knee. During
the knee bending the heel of the rear foot must be kept in contact with
the floor and the knee must be kept straight. The right calf muscles
are stretched when the right foot is in the rear position, and the left
when the left foot occupies this position.

Zinc oxide strapping

Four strips of 2 in. zinc oxide adhesive plaster are moulded round the
leg so that they cover the injured area and extend above and below it
(Fig. 108, p. 167). The two straps for the upper part of the leg should
be about 18 in. long; the other two should be about 16 in. long.

Position of player. The strapping is applied with the player in half-lying;
a folded pillow is placed under the thigh, so as to flex the knee and
leave a deep space under the leg.

Technique of strapping. The straps are moulded round the leg from
behind, the same technique being used as described on p. 163 for thigh
strapping.

Application of 1st strap. The first strap is applied behind the leg, well
below the injured area. The inner end is taken across the front of the
leg in a slanting direction; the outer end is then carried across it. *See*
Fig. 107.

Application of 2nd and 3rd straps. The second and third straps are
applied in the same manner as the first strap, but each strap overlaps
the previous one by about a third of its width. (Fig. 107.)

Application of 4th strap. The fourth strap must be applied slightly
differently from the other straps, because of the shape of the upper
calf. It is placed horizontally behind the calf, and the main portion
moulded to the shape of the muscles; the lower edge overlaps the
previous strap by about a third of its width. The inner end is brought

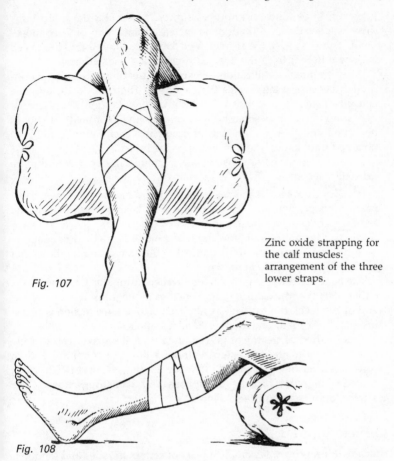

Fig. 107

Zinc oxide strapping for
the calf muscles:
arrangement of the three
lower straps.

Fig. 108

Outer aspect of the completed strapping. The fourth strap is
arranged horizontally behind the calf.

round to the front of the leg, the therapist allowing it to follow its own
inclination as regards direction. The outer end is treated in the same
way, so that it overlaps the inner end. Fig. 108 shows the completed
strapping.

Bruising or haematoma of thigh

A haematoma of the thigh is treated in the same way as a muscle tear
(pp. 158–163). It generally responds to treatment in about 7 to 10 days.

Haematoma complicated by traumatic ossification (p. 157)

Knee movement returns rapidly after a straightforward haematoma.
When the haematoma is complicated by traumatic ossification,

however, knee function improves slowly for about 4 days; after this there is a secondary stiffness and increased limitation of knee movement. There is also a hard, solid 'feel' about the injured muscle, which is quite different from the 'feel' of a recovering haematoma.

When traumatic ossification is suspected, treatment must be discontinued, because it aggravates the condition. The club doctor must be consulted, and if he decides that traumatic ossification is present he may prescribe rest or some form of conservative treatment. It should be noted that X-ray evidence of traumatic ossification cannot be obtained until about 3 to 6 weeks after the injury.

The following type of conservative treatment has been found to be extremely useful.

Immobilization of knee. The knee is immobilized in extension by a viscopaste bandage, which is applied over a thick layer of cotton wool. The bandage covers the upper two-thirds of the leg and the lower two-thirds of the thigh. A simple spiral technique is used in bandaging, and the upper turns are applied direct to the skin of the thigh, so that the bandage does not slip down.

The bandage is left in position for a week; during this time the player either rests the injured limb completely or reduces his activity. At the end of the week the bandage is removed; active knee flexion is measured and recorded, and another bandage applied.

This method of treatment is continued until the player can actively flex the knee to the full extent without pain. The condition is then considered as being resolved. If X-ray findings support this view, exercises to redevelop the quadriceps and hamstring muscles are started; light training is also allowed.

Severe injuries

Severe injuries include complete tears of certain muscles and tendons. The muscles most commonly injured in this way are the rectus femoris, the hamstrings and the calf; usually the tear occurs at the musculotendinous junction. Tendons which are sometimes completely torn include the extensor tendon of the quadriceps muscle at the upper border of the patella, the adductor longus tendon in the crutch, and the Achilles tendon.

Treatment. A ruptured muscle is either treated by surgery or by the methods previously described for partial tears (pp. 158–163). Neither operative repair nor conservative treatment restores the original power to the muscle, and the player is unlikely to be good enough for first-class athletics or play.

A tendon which is completely ruptured is repaired by surgery. The joint on which it acts is immobilized in a plaster cast for several weeks. When the cast is removed exercises are given to redevelop the muscles and restore joint mobility.

Part 4
Treatment of trunk and neck injuries

Chapter 13
Injuries of the trunk and neck

Injuries of the trunk and neck may be divided into four main groups: (1) Displacement or prolapse of one of the intervertebral discs ('slipped' disc); (2) Muscle strains, tears and bruises; (3) Sprains of ligaments, and (4) Rib fractures. Fibrositis or muscular rheumatism must also be mentioned in connection with injuries of the trunk and neck, because the condition frequently occurs after a muscle strain or tear.

Prolapsed lumbar intervertebral disc
'Slipped' Disc

The spinal discs. The spinal discs consist of thick fibrous pads which link together the bodies of the vertebrae, as shown in Fig. 109. They act as shock absorbers, and enable all kinds of spinal movements to be performed without damage or discomfort.

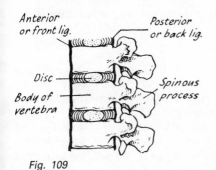

Fig. 109

Side view of lumbar vertebrae, showing spinal discs. Discs cut to show pulpy cores.

Each disc consists of two parts: an outer ring of fibro-cartilage, and an inner core of pulpy jelly-like material. (Fig. 110.)

The discs are not only blended with the bones of the spinal column, but also with the two broad, ribbon-like ligaments which lie on the front and back surfaces of the vertebral bodies, as shown in Fig. 109, p. 171.

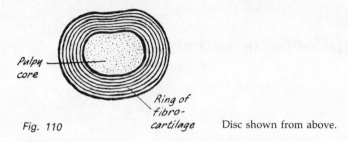

Pulpy core

Ring of fibro- cartilage

Fig. 110   Disc shown from above.

Behind the discs and the vertebral bodies lies the spinal canal. (Fig. 111.) It contains the nerve roots which pass down from the spinal cord. These nerves branch out of the canal in pairs, lying behind the discs, as shown in Fig. 111. Outside the canal the nerves descend to supply the structures of the lower limb.

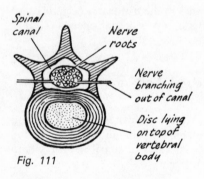

Spinal canal

Nerve roots

Nerve branching out of canal

Disc lying on top of vertebral body

Fig. 111

Diagram of lumbar vertebra, seen from above, to show position of disc and nerve roots.

Injuries to the discs

Injuries of the lumbar discs are common. The discs between the 4th and 5th lumbar vertebrae and between the 5th lumbar and the 1st sacral vertebrae are those most often affected.

A frequent cause of injury is lifting a heavy weight with the back rounded, instead of the spine being kept straight. Overstressing the final degrees of forward bending movements of the spine is another common cause of injury. This can happen when the toe-touching type of limbering-up exercises are carried out too enthusiastically at the start of the season, especially when the hamstrings are short. Other causes of injury include flexion and rotation strains of the spine (for example, bending down with a twist of the trunk to pick up an object from the floor), and sneezing while in a bent position.

Forcing the spine into the bent position compresses the front parts of the lumbar discs, and the pulpy cores are squeezed backwards, as shown in Fig. 112. If the force used is severe, one or more of the discs may be nipped and damaged, as explained later.

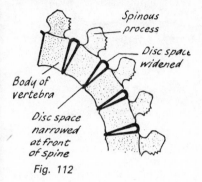

Fig. 112

To show how the shape of the discs alters when the spine is bent forwards.

Symptoms. A lumbar disc injury gives rise to pain in the lower back, buttock and back of the thigh. The pain may occur immediately after the injury or begin gradually a few hours or days later. Often the pain starts in the lower back ('lumbago') and spreads down to the buttock and thigh (sciatica). Sometimes, however, the pain starts in the leg and spreads to the back. In a few cases the symptoms may be confined to the back and never radiate to the leg.

The pain varies from a dull ache to a stabbing, neuralgic pain. When the pain is very bad all ordinary movements of the spine are impossible, and the player feels that his back is completely 'locked'. Coughing and sneezing make the pain worse, and shifting from one position to another – as in getting up from a chair – is often an agonizing experience.

Mechanism of injury. When the front part of a disc is nipped or compressed by a flexion strain (*see* Fig. 112) the pulpy core is pressed forcibly against its fibrous coverings; in severe strains the pulp is squeezed out of the centre of the disc (Fig. 113) rather like toothpaste being pressed out of a tube. In less severe strains the disc wall bulges backwards, as shown in Fig. 114.

If the displacement of the disc is small the protrusion bulges against the sensitive posterior ligament (Fig. 115) and pain is felt in the back. If it is large the protrusion breaks through the posterior ligament and impinges upon one of the spinal nerves, so that it is stretched, as shown in Fig. 116; this causes sciatic pain.

When the back part of a disc is nipped, as sometimes occurs when the spine is bent backwards violently, the pulpy core is displaced

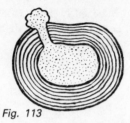

Fig. 113

A disc after a severe nipping strain: the pulp has broken through the fibrous ring.

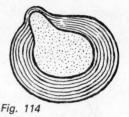

Fig. 114

A disc after a less severe strain: the fibrous ring bulges at its weakest part.

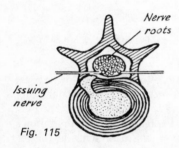

Fig. 115

To show the effect of a small backward displacement of a lumbar disc: the protrusion bulges against the sensitive posterior spinal ligament.

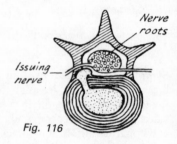

Fig. 116

When a large backward displacement of a lumbar disc occurs the protrusion breaks through the posterior ligament and impinges upon one of the spinal nerves.

forwards. Usually this type of displacement does not produce symptoms, because the pulp merely pushes the front ligament of the spine forwards and there are no nerve trunks in this area to give rise to pain. *See* Fig. 109, p. 171.

Natural healing. Once the pulpy core of a disc has forced its way through its fibrous coverings it is extremely unlikely that it can return to its original place again. Over a period of several months the pulp shrinks gradually and the tension on the spinal nerve is relieved. This explains why many disc injuries recover slowly without treatment. A bulge in the disc coverings also tends to shrink gradually.

Treatment

Treatment for lumbar disc injuries takes two forms: conservative or non-operative treatment, and operative treatment (removal of the protruding portion of the disc). Conservative treatment is successful in relieving the symptoms in at least nineteen out of every twenty cases, and consists of: (1) Rest in bed, with or without spinal traction, (2) Plaster-of-paris jacket, (3) Intermittent spinal traction, and (4) Spinal manipulation.

Conservative treatment

Rest in bed for 3 weeks. The player lies flat on his back on a firm mattress, and is not allowed to bend his spine or to get out of bed. Boards are placed under the mattress to prevent the trunk from sagging.

Some orthopaedic surgeons advise the player to rest completely during the period in bed; others like him to practise exercises to strengthen the back muscles.

When the player is allowed up he practises exercises to strengthen the extensor and rotator muscles of the spine. *See* specimen exercises, p. 177. Forward bending exercises are not allowed. Generally the surgeon advises the wearing of a broad webbing support round the lumbar spine and hips; its main purpose is to remind the player to keep the spine erect when sitting and standing, and not to let it bend forwards.

Rest in bed with spinal traction. The player rests in bed for about three weeks, as previously described, but a constant traction pull of about 8 lb. is applied to each leg by means of strapping and a simple weight-and-pulley circuit. The traction is continued until the acute pain has subsided; it is then discontinued (or the weight reduced gradually) and the player rests freely in bed. A supporting belt is generally worn when he is allowed up, and trunk exercises are practised as previously described. *See* specimen exercises, p. 177.

Plaster-of-paris jacket. An alternative to the previous treatments consists of the player wearing a plaster-of-paris jacket for several weeks. The jacket fits snugly round the hips and lower half of the trunk; it rests the lumbar spine and prevents it from bending forwards. While wearing the jacket the player maintains the strength of his back muscles by practising the extension exercises described on. p. 177.

Intermittent spinal traction. Sometimes when the pain is not too severe the surgeon recommends intermittent spinal traction. The player attends the hospital physiotherapy department each day, and traction is applied to the spine for a period of about 20 to 30 minutes; a traction force of up to 180 lb. is used. A special traction couch is necessary, but the treatment is by no means as drastic or uncomfortable as it sounds. Intermittent traction is usually given over a period of about 2 weeks.

Spinal manipulation. Occasionally the surgeon manipulates the player's spine; usually a general anaesthetic is used to secure complete muscular relaxation.

When manipulation succeeds in relieving the symptoms of a disc injury it is probably because the displaced portion of the disc has been shifted from the area where it was impinging on a spinal nerve or pressing against the posterior ligament, to an area where it is relatively free.

Resuming training. Training is not resumed until the surgeon is satisfied that the pain has cleared up completely and the back muscles are strong and acting normally. No hard and fast times can be suggested, but after rest in bed (with or without traction) training is often started about 4 to 6 weeks after getting up. Less time is usually necessary between the termination of the other conservative treatments and the start of training.

Operative treatment

An operation to remove the displaced disc material is known as a *laminectomy*. It is only performed when conservative measures have been given a fair trial and have failed to relieve severe sciatic pain. Sciatic pain can be so excruciating that it prevents sleep and leads to a marked deterioration of the general health.

After the operation the patient is returned to his ward from the operating theatre in a side-lying position with the hips and knees flexed to about 45°. This is maintained for at least 24 hours, the position being changed by the nursing staff from right to left, and *vice versa*, at two-hour intervals. A firm pillow is positioned between the knees.

After the second post-operative day the patient is allowed to take up a back-lying position in bed. From then on his resting position varies between back lying and side lying with knees crooked.

During this period the patient is encouraged to carry out simple breathing, ankle and foot exercises to prevent post-operative respiratory and circulatory complications.

Sitting. The patient is allowed to sit out in a suitable chair, at his bedside, for short periods between the second and fifth post-operative day. He is discharged home when the sutures have been removed on the tenth or twelfth post-operative day.

Back exercises in bed. From about the third to the tenth or twelfth post-operative day the patient is generally allowed to carry out small-range exercises to maintain the strength of the muscles of the thoracolumbar spine. Examples include: (1) Lying, slight chest raising (arching of the spine); (2) Lying, opposite arm and leg downpressing into the bed; and (3) Lying face downwards, raising each leg backwards, in turn, about 30°. *No* forward bending movements of the spine are allowed at this stage.

Exercises after tenth or twelfth post-operative day. When he has been discharged from hospital it is most important that the patient continues with exercises which have the effect of strengthening the extensor muscles of the thoracolumbar spine, and increasing the mobility of the spinal joints. Forward bending movements of the spine are gradually introduced, but no *forced* flexion exercises (e.g. toe-touching with straight knees) are permitted.

Suitable forward bending movements include: (a) Side lying, with knees and hips flexed to about 45°, bending up the knees to the chest, and (b) Sitting on a firm chair, with hands resting on thighs, allowing the spine to bend forwards in a relaxed manner.

It is also essential for the patient to learn how to guard his back against stresses and strains which may result in injury. Some of the practical points for him to observe are listed here: (a) When lifting any heavy weight from a low level keep the weight close to the body, with the back straight. Use the hips and knees to do the work of lifting, rather than the back; (b) Avoid any sustained bending forwards; (c) *Avoid, at all costs, a combination of lifting and twisting with a bent back.* This exposes the spine to severe mechanical stresses, and may well injure the joints; (d) Sit with adequate back support, and always remember to stand 'tall' and avoid 'slumping'.

Resuming training. The player is usually allowed to resume training about two months after the operation. The time factor depends entirely on the opinion of the surgeon.

Spinal exercises

Extension exercises
1. Lying face downwards, arms to sides, palms upwards: bend trunk backwards while turning the arms outwards. (Fig. 117.)
2. As previous exercise, but the player's legs are fixed by the feet being tucked under the wall-bars or some heavy object. (Fig. 118.)
3. As Ex. 1, but as the trunk is bent backwards one of the legs is raised backwards as far as possible. (Fig. 119.) Each leg is moved in turn.
4. Lying on back with arms folded across the chest, legs astride and knees bent to about 90°: press up to high Wrestler's Bridge. (Fig. 120.) A progression of this exercise consists of pressing up to a low Wrestler's Bridge; the starting position is the same as for the high Bridge, but the knees are only slightly flexed.

Rotation exercises
1. Lying on back with legs astride, arms to sides, palms downwards:

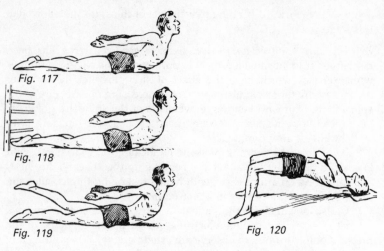

Figs. 117–120. A series of exercises to strengthen the back muscles.

(a) Turn trunk to left, at the same time reaching across the chest with the right arm; (b) Return to starting position; (c) Turn trunk turning to right, at the same time reaching across chest with left arm, and (d) Return to starting position.
2. Lying face downwards, arms to sides, and feet fixed by wall-bars or some heavy object: (a) Bend trunk backwards, at the same time attempting to look over the right shoulder as much as possible; (b) Return to starting position; (c) Bend trunk backwards, at the same time looking over the left shoulder, and (d) Return to starting position.

Exercise technique. The exercises should be performed smoothly and fairly slowly; at the end of each complete movement the player should relax for a few moments. The rotation exercises should be 'spaced' between the extension exercises to avoid over-fatiguing the back muscles.

The player should exercise for about 20 to 30 minutes, two or three times daily, if possible.

Prolapsed cervical (neck) disc

Displacement of intervertebral disc material in the neck is much less common than it is in the lumbar spine. When it occurs it is usually as a result of some jarring or twisting strain of the neck. At the time the injury may appear to be slight, and there may not be any immediate effects. Hours or days later an acute 'stiff neck' develops; later pain radiates over the shoulder and down the arm.

Treatment. When the symptoms are slight, hot packs, ultrasound or interferential therapy may be used. Gentle massage to the neck extensor muscles is also helpful. In the more severe cases the neck may have to be rested in a supporting plastic collar for about 6 weeks. Sometimes rest in bed with continuous head traction is used for 2 to 3 weeks as an alternative.

Operative removal of cervical disc protrusions is seldom carried out.

Muscle strains, tears and bruises

The muscles most commonly involved are the spinal extensors (particularly those of the lumbar region), the abdominal muscles, and the muscles lying between the ribs.

Treatment is the same as that described for injuries of the thigh and leg muscles (p. 158), with the exception that it is not practicable to strap the muscles or apply pressure bandages.

Possibility of inguinal hernia (rupture). It is important to realize that pain in the lower abdominal muscles, close to the crutch, may not be due to a muscle injury, but may be a symptom of an inguinal hernia or rupture. Often it is extremely difficult to differentiate between the two conditions, and medical advice is essential.

Sprains of ligaments

The ligaments most frequently sprained are those of the lumbar spine and neck (pp. 91 and 92). Treatment follows the lines suggested for sprains of the ankle and knee, with the exception that it is not practicable to use pressure bandages and strapping supports. Neither can massage be used because of the inaccessibility of the ligaments; the supraspinous ligament (which connects the tips of the spinous processes from the 7th cervical vertebra to the sacrum), however, can be treated.

Disc damage complicating muscular and ligamentous injuries of the lumbar spine

A muscular or ligamentous injury of the lumbar spine often gives rise to the same type of low back pain or 'lumbago' which characterizes an injury of one of the lumbar intervertebral discs (p. 172). If the injury does not respond satisfactorily to treatment, or is complicated later by a radiating pain in one of the buttocks and down the back of the thigh, medical advice should be sought, because the symptoms suggest a lumbar disc displacement or prolapse. *See* p. 172.

Rib fractures

Fractures of the ribs occur fairly often, especially in body-contact sports. Generally only one of the ribs is involved. Localized acute pain over a rib, particularly on deep inspiration, suggests a fracture. The player should be seen by the club doctor as soon as possible.

Treatment. After the fracture has been proved by an X-ray examination the doctor may suggest that the injured area of the chest should be strapped firmly for about 14 days; on the other hand he may decide that support is not necessary; much depends on the degree of pain felt by the player.

Strapping. Two methods of support are used:
1. The chest is encircled by two or three overlapping turns of 3 in. elastoplast, the strapping being centred over the injured area. When the elastoplast is being applied the player should be told to breathe out as much as possible.
2. Two or three strips of 2 in. zinc oxide adhesive plaster are applied to the injured side of the chest, so that they overlap each other slightly and cover the painful area. They should extend from the sternum in front to well beyond the midline of the back, and be arranged obliquely. As the strapping is applied the player should breathe out deeply.

Fibrositis or muscular rheumatism

Fibrositis is a term which is widely used to describe painful and tender areas in certain muscles and their overlying fascia and skin. Pain and tenderness are particularly evident when the muscles are gripped and squeezed; sometimes small, firm nodules may be felt. Joint movements are full and there are no other clinical signs.

Fibrositis occurs most frequently in relation to the muscles of the neck, shoulder-blades, lumbar and lumbosacral regions. (Fig. 121.)

Causes. The causes are not fully understood, but various explanations have been suggested:

1. Draughts, chills, exposure, damp and cold.
2. Over-use and strains of muscles, tearing of some of their fibres, and other injuries.
3. Worry and late nights.
4. A septic focus. Often the focus is obvious – e.g. septic teeth – but sometimes it is extremely difficult to find.

Treatment. When the condition is acute and extremely painful the part should be rested, and some form of heat therapy used – hot baths, packs, infra-red radiation or short-wave therapy. Massage should be

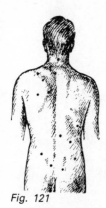

Main areas of fibrositic pain.

Fig. 121

given when the player can tolerate it. The tight skin over the fibrositic areas must be loosened thoroughly by skin rollings and kneadings, and the tender areas in the muscles treated by deep transverse and circular frictions.

The massage will be extremely painful – particularly during the first few treatments – and the player must be warned beforehand about this. He must be told that unless the massage is deep it will be a complete waste of time. Usually treatment can only be given on alternate days because of the painful reaction.

Exercises. After the massage the player should exercise the affected muscles to improve their blood supply. 'Warming-up' mobility movements should be used. It cannot be too strongly emphasized that exercises are of no value whatever in the treatment of fibrositis unless they are associated with deep massage.

Part 5
Treatment of upper limb injuries

Chapter 14
Injuries of the fingers, wrist and elbow

Sprains of the fingers, wrist and elbow are treated in much the same way as sprains of the ankle and knee (pp. 113 to 133), with the exception that elastoplast or crêpe bandage supports are used in place of pressure bandages in the early stage of treatment; a pressure bandage might restrict the circulation through the injured part because the fascial membrane which covers the soft tissues of the upper limb is not as thick and unyielding as that of the lower limb.

For definition and degrees of sprain *see* p. 112.

Sprains of the fingers and thumb

Sprains of the fingers and thumb occur chiefly in contact sports, particularly rugby, boxing and wrestling. The medial and lateral ligaments of the knuckle or metacarpo-phalangeal joints (Fig. 122) are frequently injured, usually as a result of a sideways or backwards strain. Swelling of the joint is accompanied by pain on movement, especially on attempted gripping. The joint is also tender on sideways pressure.

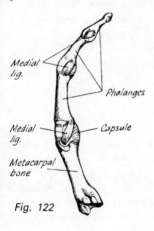

Medial lig.

Phalanges

Medial lig.

Capsule

Metacarpal bone

Fig. 122   Inner aspect of the joints of a finger.

Sprains of the fingers and thumb are often regarded as trivial injuries. This is a mistake, because if they are not treated carefully they can give rise to persistent swelling and pain over a period of several weeks or months. It is particularly important to avoid moving the injured joint passively, and massage is best avoided.

Treatment

Immediately after the injury the hand should be rested for about 24 hours; there seems little to be gained by strapping the injured joint, but this may be done. After the period of rest a variety of physical treatments may be used: ultrasonic therapy (with injured hand immersed in an arm-bath or deep bowl, so that water forms the couplant between treatment head and skin), pulsed short-wave therapy or paraffin wax. Contrast bathing is also helpful.

Active movements of the fingers and thumb are started within a pain-free range, and the player should be encouraged to use the hand as normally as possible. Early exercises should include 'making a fist' and relaxing the muscles slowly, and straightening the fingers and thumb to the full extent and allowing the muscles to slacken off slowly. As the injury improves, the amount of exercise given should be increased. Helpful exercises include squeezing a sorbo-rubber ball and rolling up a sheet of newspaper, or an unrolled crêpe bandage, into a tight ball in the palm of the hand without assistance from the sound hand.

Later, simple stick exercises (using a light broomstick) provide excellent functional movement for the hand as a whole, and help to develop the grip. Useful exercises include: (a) Standing (holding a stick at arm's length, with one hand placed immediately above the other), and causing the stick to 'travel' upwards and downwards by alternating the position of the hands and (b) Standing (with arms stretched forwards at shoulder level, and one hand grasping the middle of a vertically held stick), and throwing stick rhythmically from hand to hand.

The majority of simple sprains of the fingers and thumb clear up within about 10 days. The more severe types of sprain, however, may need a much longer period of treatment.

Resuming training. At the end of about 10 days' treatment the injured ligament is tested passively (p. 228); if the result is satisfactory, training is resumed. If the player is returning to a strenuous game, such as rugby football, it is a wise precaution to strap the injured joint before each training session and game (p. 22). When a finger has been sprained it is usually sufficient to strap it *loosely* to the adjacent sound finger with narrow strips of zinc oxide plaster; the fingers should be strapped in the relaxed position of rest, and *not* in extension. When the thumb has been sprained a figure-of-eight strapping of zinc oxide plaster is used, as described here.

Figure-of-eight strapping for thumb

The thumb is strapped by three pieces of zinc oxide adhesive plaster, each piece measuring 18 × 1 in.; the straps are arranged in such a way that they prevent the thumb from being forced back into hyperextension. The strapping is completed by a piece of zinc oxide plaster about 10 × 2 in.

The long straps are applied with the thumb in the position shown in Fig. 123 (abduction combined with some opposition); the elbow is bent to about 90°, and the forearm is held with the palm facing inwards and the thumb uppermost.

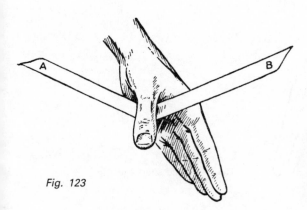

Fig. 123

The start of the figure-of-eight strapping for the thumb.

Technique
1. The centre of the first strap is placed round the palmar surface of the thumb, close to the cleft, as shown in Fig. 123. The inner end of the strap (A) is then carried outwards over the knuckle joint of the thumb, over the back of the wrist, and round to the front of the joint. The outer end of the strap (B) is taken inwards across the knuckle joint, and then carried downwards over the front of the wrist, under it, and round to the back of the joint. Fig. 124 shows the first strap in position.
2. The second strap is applied in the same manner as the previous one, but it overlaps it by about two-thirds of its width.
3. The third strap is applied in the same way as the second strap.
4. The broad strap of zinc oxide plaster is placed over the front of the wrist; the ends are then folded, in turn, round the back of the joint so that they cross each other. Fig. 125 shows the completed strapping.

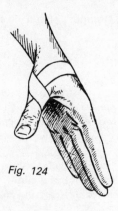

Fig. 124

The first strap in position.

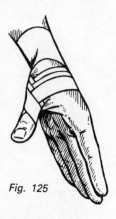

Fig. 125

The completed strapping.

Ruptured ligaments

A complete tear of a finger or thumb ligament is uncommon. When it occurs the joint is unstable and weak, and there is unnatural mobility. Treatment consists of fixing the finger or thumb (in the position of rest) in a plaster cast for about 3 to 4 weeks. When the cast is removed exercises are used to restore the mobility of the injured joint and to strengthen the muscles which act on it

Sprain of the wrist

In general, sprain of the wrist is a relatively uncommon injury. When it occurs it is usually as the result of a fall on the outstretched hand, and the front ligament of the joint (Fig. 126) is injured. The back ligament (Fig. 46, p. 94) is sometimes sprained by the wrist being forced beyond the normal range of flexion. Swelling and tenderness of the joint are the main symptoms.

The injury must be seen as soon as possible by the club doctor, because what appears to be a simple sprain of the wrist may well be

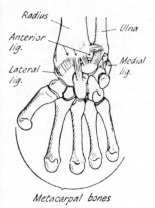

Fig. 126

Diagrammatic impression of the ligaments of the right wrist: front or palmar view.

a fracture of the carpal scaphoid bone (Fig. 45, p. 94). A scaphoid fracture can only be detected by X-rays, and unless it is treated correctly (by the wrist being fixed in a plaster cast for several weeks) it seldom unites. *See* also p. 95.

Treatment

For the first 24 hours after the injury the wrist should be supported by a firm crêpe bandage, as described on p. 190, and the forearm and hand rested completely; a triangular arm sling is sometimes used.

After the period of rest a variety of treatments may be used: interferential therapy, short-wave therapy or paraffin wax. Contrast bathing is also of value. Active movements of the wrist, fingers and forearm joints are started within a pain-free range of movement, and progressed gradually. The supporting bandage is replaced after treatment, and the player is encouraged to move the fingers as much as possible during the day. It is a good plan if he carries a sorbo-rubber ball around with him and squeezes it at frequent intervals; a small roll of sponge rubber is sometimes found to be more useful for gripping movements than the ball.

Resuming training. The symptoms usually subside in about 7 to 10 days. The injured ligament is then tested passively (p. 228); if the result is satisfactory, training is resumed. At each training session the wrist must be supported by an elastoplast strapping, as described on

p. 191. The wrist must also be strapped in the same way when the player returns to the game. *See* p. 22.

Crêpe bandage support for wrist

A 3 in. crêpe bandage is used. It is applied with the player's elbow bent and the forearm turned over so that the palm faces downwards. If the front ligament of the wrist is injured the wrist is bandaged in the *neutral* position, as shown in Fig. 127; if the back ligament is involved the wrist is bandaged in the extended position. In this way an attempt is made to keep the injured ligament in a relaxed position.

The bandage is applied reasonably tightly, a firm degree of tension being exerted on each turn. Care must be taken not to pull the bandage too tight as it is carried round the cleft of the thumb.

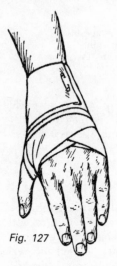

Fig. 127   Crêpe bandage support for
                               wrist.

Technique

1. The free end of the bandage is placed on the thumb side of the wrist and a couple of turns taken round it.
2. The bandage is taken downwards and outwards to the metacarpal bone of the little finger, and then carried under the palm to the cleft of the thumb.
3. The bandage is passed upwards and outwards over the back of the hand so that it crosses the previous turn.
4. The bandage is passed under the wrist and the two previous turns are repeated; the new turns overlap the previous turns.
5. Three spiral turns of bandage are taken round the wrist and forearm in such a way that they almost overlap each other. The bandage is then cut and finished off as shown in Fig. 127.

Elastoplast support for wrist

The wrist is strapped with 3 in. elastoplast, the bandaging technique previously described being followed, with the exception that the strapping is not taken over the cleft of the thumb. Instead the thumb is enclosed in a slot, about 2 in. long, which is cut in the strapping, as shown in Fig. 128.

To finish the support the cut end of the strapping is covered with a piece of zinc oxide adhesive plaster to prevent it from wrinkling up.

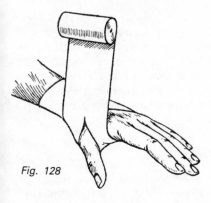

Fig. 128

When the wrist is strapped with elastoplast the thumb is enclosed in a slot cut in the strapping.

Sprain of the elbow

Sprain of the elbow is uncommon. When it occurs it is usually because of a strain which forces the joint into hyperextension and some degree of sideways movement. Generally the medial or lateral ligament (Figs. 48 and 49, p. 96) is involved. The joint becomes painful and swollen, and there is tenderness on sideways pressure.

The injury must be seen as soon as possible by the club doctor, because it may be associated with a disturbance of the periosteal covering of the bones on the front of the joint. This may lead to the formation of bony outgrowths which seriously interfere with the function of the joint. *See* Traumatic ossification, pp. 144 and 157.

Treatment

The forearm is supported by a triangular sling and the elbow rested for about 48 hours. At the end of this time pulsed short-wave therapy or interferential therapy is given.

The player is encouraged to flex and extend the elbow *actively* within a pain-free range of movement several times during the treatment period. Finger, wrist and shoulder movements are allowed, provided they do not throw any strain on the elbow. The sling is reapplied after treatment; it is worn for about 4 or 5 days.

No attempt should be made to massage the elbow or increase its range of movement by passive stretching. If traumatic ossification has occurred both these measures will aggravate the condition.

Progression. If progress is not satisfactory treatment should be discontinued, the joint rested, and the club doctor consulted. If progress is satisfactory, however, the range and strength of the elbow movements may be increased gradually. Very strong exercises which have a stretching effect on the joint (such as 'pull-ups' from a beam) should not be given for several weeks.

Resuming training. Treatment is continued until the elbow can be used normally; usually this is in about 10 or 14 days, provided that there are no complications. The injured ligament is then tested (p. 97); if the result is satisfactory, training is resumed. At each training session the elbow must be supported by an elastoplast strapping, as described below. The elbow is strapped in the same way when the player returns to the game. *See* p. 22.

Elastoplast strapping: divergent spica

The elbow is strapped with 3 in. elastoplast, a divergent spica technique being used. *See* Fig. 130, p. 193. The strapping supports the elbow firmly, especially in a sideways direction, and allows wide-range bending and stretching movements.

The spica is applied with the player's elbow bent to about 45° and the forearm turned over so that the palm faces downwards. A firm degree of tension should be exerted on each turn of strapping as it is carried round the joint. The turns on the front of the elbow should be made to overlap each other as much as possible, so as to facilitate movement.

Technique

1. The free end of the strapping is placed on the upper side of the joint with the roll of strapping held close to the 'point' of the elbow. A couple of turns of strapping are taken round the joint. (Fig. 129.)

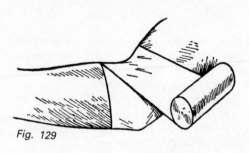

Fig. 129

Elastoplast support for elbow: the start of the spica technique.

2. The strapping is carried in a curved direction above the 'point' of the elbow, so that it covers the upper half of the previous turns. The free end is brought down level with the previous turns on the under side of the joint. The strapping is then passed in front of the joint over the previous turns.

3. The same process is repeated, but the strapping is taken below the 'point' of the elbow.

4. The strapping is taken above the 'point' of the elbow so that over three-quarters of the upper curved turn is covered. It is then taken in front of the joint.

5. The strapping is taken below the 'point' of the elbow in the same manner.

6. The strapping is brought in front of the joint, taken to the upper side, and cut. A small piece of zinc oxide adhesive plaster is placed over the end to prevent it from wrinkling up. (Fig. 130.)

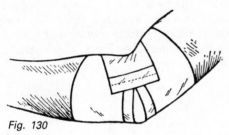

The completed strapping.

Fig. 130

Chapter 15
Tennis and golfer's elbow

'Tennis elbow'

'Tennis elbow' is a common condition which is characterized by pain and tenderness over the outer side of the elbow at the site of origin of the extensor muscles of the wrist (lateral epicondyle: Fig. 131); the pain often radiates down the back of the forearm. It is caused by overuse and strain of the forearm muscles, and is particularly likely to follow sports and occupations which call for an excessive amount of forearm rotation and gripping, such as tennis, fly-fishing, weight-lifting, massage and hedge-clipping.

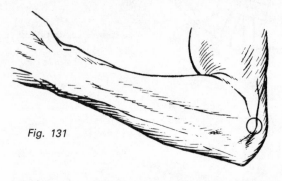

Fig. 131

Outer aspect of arm and forearm showing position of lateral epicondyle.

Doctors are divided in their opinion as to the exact nature of the injury. Some consider it to be a tearing of a few fibres of the wrist extensor muscles at their origin (Fig. 131); others think that it is an inflammation of the periosteal covering of the lateral epicondyle, due to repeated irritation by muscle-pulls.

'Tennis elbow' usually clears up without treatment over a period of several months; sometimes the symptoms persist for up to 2 years or more. The player is seldom willing to wait for the condition to subside spontaneously, however, because he is unable to play with the affected arm; any attempt to do so causes pain. Once the symptoms have subsided they do not usually recur, even if the game or occupation which was originally responsible is undertaken again.

Treatment

Many different types of conservative treatment are used for 'tennis elbow', which indicates that it is a difficult condition to deal with. Electrotherapy measures include ultrasound, pulsed short-wave and interferential therapy. Other treatments range from strapping, injections of novocaine or hydrocortisone, manipulation of the elbow, and immobilization of the wrist in a plaster cast, to deep massage by transverse frictions. Operative treatment is sometimes advised in cases of severe disability which do not respond to conservative treatment.

The most useful forms of therapy appear to be manipulation, transverse frictions and immobilization of the wrist. The actual choice of treatment (and its subsequent success) depends entirely on a correct assessment of the injury, i.e. whether it is a pure muscle tear, a periostitis, or a combination of both. This requires considerable experience and judgement, and the club doctor generally considers it advisable to consult an orthopaedic surgeon who has specialized in the treatment of soft-tissue injuries.

Manipulation. The elbow is manipulated under general anaesthesia. Active elbow and wrist exercises are practised as soon as the player regains consciousness, and are continued for several days. The exercises must include movements which put the wrist extensor muscles on the stretch.

Transverse frictions. Deep friction is applied to the front part of the lateral epicondyle (Fig. 131); during treatment the extensor muscles of the wrist must be kept on the stretch. To achieve this the operator keeps the player's wrist flexed and the forearm pronated (palm downward position).

Immobilization of wrist. The wrist is immobilized in full extension in a plaster cast for about 6 weeks. The elbow is not included in the cast.

'Golfer's elbow'

'Golfer's elbow' is a similar condition to 'tennis elbow', but pain and tenderness are localized to the inner side of the elbow, just below the medial epicondyle (Fig. 132). It is caused by a strain of the long flexor muscles of the wrist close to their site of origin.

Unlike 'tennis elbow', the disability does not clear up spontaneously. Treatment by deep massage, however, is extremely effective and brings about recovery in three or four weeks. Treatment is painful and should only be given on alternate days.

Treatment technique. Transverse friction is applied to the tender area of the elbow with the wrist flexor muscles on the stretch. The player is treated in half-lying (Fig. 61, p. 114), with the upper limb supported by a pillow; to keep the wrist flexors stretched the elbow and wrist are maintained in extension and the forearm in supination (palm upward position).

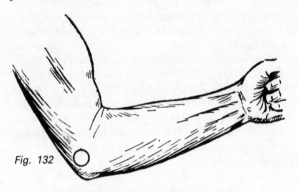

Fig. 132

Inner aspect of arm and forearm showing position of medial epicondyle.

Chapter 16

Injuries of the shoulder and shoulder-girdle

Common soft-tissue injuries of the shoulder region include: (1) Subluxation and dislocation of the acromio-clavicular joint, (2) Dislocation of the shoulder joint, (3) Sub-deltoid bursitis, and (4) Strains and tears of the 'rotator' cuff.

Acromio-clavicular injuries

The acromio-clavicular joint (Fig. 50, p. 98) is often injured as a result of a fall or a blow on the point of the shoulder; horsemen and rugby players are frequent sufferers. If the injury is confined to a tearing of the acromio-clavicular ligament, subluxation (or partial dislocation) of the joint occurs, as shown in Fig. 133. If there is a complete rupture of both the acromio-clavicular and coraco-clavicular ligaments (Fig. 134) the acromio-clavicular joint is dislocated.

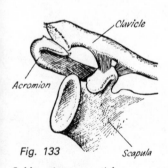

Fig. 133

Subluxation or partial dislocation of the right acromio-clavicular joint.

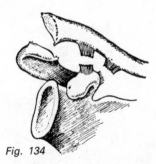

Fig. 134

Dislocation of the right acromio-clavicular joint.

Acromio-clavicular subluxation

The outer end of the clavicle is raised a little higher than the acromion, as shown in Fig. 133. Sometimes the displacement is obscured by swelling, but the injury is revealed by tenderness localized to the joint line.

Treatment. The joint must be maintained in a corrected position by means of a strapping support which passes over the shoulder girdle and under the flexed elbow. (Figs. 136 and 137, p. 199.) The strapping is worn for about 3 weeks.

When the strapping is removed exercises are given to restore the mobility of the shoulder and elbow joints, and to strengthen the muscles. Excellent functional results follow this méthod of treatment, although a slight upward displacement of the clavicle always occurs.

Strapping technique. The elbow is flexed to just over a right angle, and a pad of cotton wool placed over the shoulder-girdle. The free end of a roll of 3 in. elastoplast is applied over the inner aspect of the clavicle and chest, as shown in Fig. 135. The strapping is then carried backwards over the shoulder-girdle and down behind the arm. A pad of cotton wool is placed under the forearm, close to the elbow, and the strapping is taken round it. The strapping is then passed obliquely upwards to the root of the neck, so that it crosses the starting end, and is brought down over the shoulder blade, where it is cut. (Fig. 136.) The forearm is then supported by a triangular sling. (Fig. 137.)

During the application of the strapping the humerus is pushed upwards and the clavicle pulled downwards. A second or third layer of elastoplast is sometimes added to the original strapping, because it may be stretched by the weight of the limb.

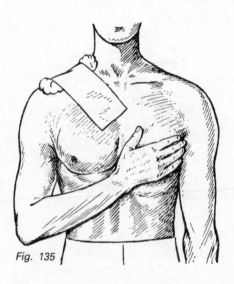

Fig. 135

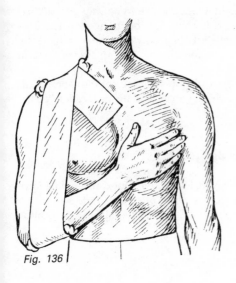

Fig. 136

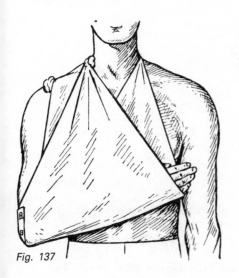

Fig. 137

Figs. 135–137. Method of holding acromio-clavicular joint in corrected position after subluxation.

Acromio-clavicular dislocation

This is a comparatively rare injury. Displacement is greater than in a subluxation, and the outer end of the clavicle rides high above the acromion. (Fig. 134, p. 197.)

Treatment. The injury is usually treated in the same way as a subluxation, but the strapping support is worn for about 6 weeks. The ligaments re-form reasonably well, but they do not become sufficiently taut to prevent all displacement of the clavicle; the function of the arm is usually good.

Fascial reconstruction of the torn ligaments is sometimes attempted. The 'new' ligaments often stretch, however, and the dislocation recurs.

Dislocation of the shoulder joint

For a dislocation to occur in a normal shoulder joint considerable force must be applied. The injury occurs fairly often in sport. Perhaps in certain circumstances the shoulder joint is susceptible to dislocation

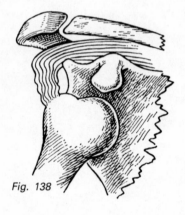

Fig. 138

Dislocation of the right shoulder joint.

because of the large head of the humerus articulating with the shallow glenoid cavity, and the lax capsule.

The strength of the shoulder joint depends largely on the power of its muscles. The mechanism of dislocation is the arrest of rotation at the shoulder joint, e.g. by a fall on the outstretched arm.

Signs. Dislocation of the shoulder joint is often overlooked. The following signs are reliable: (1) extreme pain and complete loss of function; (2) some flattening over the upper part of the shoulder; (3) the arm seems longer than the other one, and does not lie parallel with the chest wall: the elbow cannot be made to touch the side; (4) active movement of the shoulder cannot be obtained; and (5) the player leans over towards the injured side and supports the elbow.

Treatment

The club doctor should examine the player as soon as possible after the injury. An X-ray is taken to see whether there has been a fracture, and the dislocation is reduced; a general anaesthetic is usually necessary. The arm is supported by a triangular or collar-and-cuff sling.

Heat therapy. The day after reduction the shoulder is treated by infra-red radiation or short-wave diathermy;[1] the treatment is given daily for about 10 days.

Exercise therapy. Some doctors advise that the shoulder should be kept completely immobilized in the sling for about 3 weeks; static contractions of the shoulder muscles are allowed, together with exercises for the elbow, forearm, wrist and fingers. After this time shoulder exercises are started, as described here, to restore the mobility of the joint and strengthen the muscles. Other doctors permit movement of the shoulder a few days after the injury, provided a careful system of exercises is used, as described in this section.

Progressive exercises. Exercises for the shoulder should be started in the stooping position, as shown in Fig. 139, so that no strain is thrown on the torn capsule, e.g. small range flexion and extension (Fig. 139), rotation and circling. The exercises must be kept within a pain-free range of movement. After a day or so rotation of the shoulder is carried out in sitting, with the arm kept close to the side and the elbow flexed to a right angle.

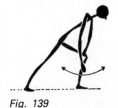

Starting position for early shoulder exercises.

Fig. 139

About 10 days from the time of injury, exercises in lying and side lying are added: (1) Lying on a couch, with the elbows fully bent, raising the arms sideways through 90°; (2) Lying on the sound side, carrying the injured arm forwards and backwards with the elbow kept straight; and (3) Lying on the sound side, with the injured arm kept close to the chest and the elbow flexed to 90°, careful inward and outward rotation of the shoulder.

[1] When the dislocation is associated with a paralysis of the deltoid muscle (*see* p. 202) heat therapy is best avoided. The skin sensation over the lower half of the deltoid will be impaired and a burn may easily occur without the player being aware of it.

When these exercises can be performed easily shoulder movements should be carried out with the player's trunk supported in an inclined position on a massage couch, as shown in Fig. 140, so that the muscles have to work harder. Progression is achieved by gradually raising the couch back until the player is exercising with the trunk in the erect position: the shoulder muscles now have the full weight of the arm to lift.

At this stage the exercises should be performed in sitting and standing, and the range of shoulder movement must be increased,

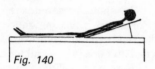

Fig. 140

Another starting position for shoulder exercises.

e.g. Arm raising sideways-upward and forwards-upward to 'stretch' position above the head. Weight (or weight-and-pulley) resisted exercises should be introduced to strengthen the shoulder muscles, special attention being paid to the abductors and outward rotators.

Normal rhythm of shoulder movement. During the exercise training great care must be taken to see that the player uses the shoulder joint in the normal manner. Often there is a tendency for him to initiate an arm raising movement by shrugging up the girdle, instead of using the shoulder joint.

Resuming training

Provided the player has regained full shoulder movement, and the muscles are as strong as those of the sound joint, training may be resumed in about 5 or 6 weeks from the time of the injury. Strapping is not required; indeed, strapping the shoulder to give support (when full joint movement is required) is a useless procedure.

Complication of dislocated shoulder

The circumflex nerve which supplies the deltoid muscle may be injured when the shoulder is dislocated, and this produces a paralysis of the muscle. The condition may be recognized by palpating the muscle belly with one hand, and asking the player to attempt an abduction movement of the shoulder against the resistance of the other hand. The player will be unable to contract the deltoid and the muscle will feel loose and flabby.

Deltoid paralysis generally clears up fairly quickly; sometimes special treatment is required.

Recurrent dislocation of the shoulder

Recurrent dislocation of the shoulder appears to be peculiar to athletes, possibly because of the degree of force which produces the initial dislocation, or exposure to repeated injury. The glenoid labrum and articular cartilage are torn from the neck of the scapula on the antero-inferior aspect, together with the insertion of the subscapularis tendon.

The recurrences are due to two factors: incomplete healing of the capsule and the specialised nature of the glenoid labrum: once torn it fails to heal. In this respect the glenoid labrum resembles the semilunar cartilages of the knee joint.

Treatment

Operative treatment is necessary to stabilise the joint, otherwise repeated dislocations will so weaken the structures that trivial twists· and strains will redisplace the articulation, e.g. putting the arm through the sleeve of a coat or shirt, raising a racquet to serve at tennis, or preparing to throw in a soccer ball.

Before the operation every effort should be made to develop the muscles acting on the joint, so as to lay the foundations for a speedy post-operative recovery.

After repair the arm is bandaged to the chest and active movement of the shoulder joint is not allowed for about 6 weeks. During this period exercises are given to maintain the joints and muscles of the shoulder-girdle, forearm, wrist and fingers.

After the removal of the fixation treatment should follow similar lines to that described for initial dislocation, p. 201.

Sub-acromial (sub-deltoid) bursitis

The sub-deltoid bursa or sac contributes largely to the smooth functioning of the shoulder joint. Fig. 141 shows its position and it is important to note that it separates the tendons of the 'rotator cuff' muscles (*see* p. 204) from the bony acromial arch. When the bursa is injured it becomes distended with synovial fluid and shoulder movement can only be carried out with considerable discomfort. Movement becomes limited, particularly abduction and outward rotation.

Sub-deltoid bursitis is usually the result of a direct blow on the shoulder, and is common in body-contact sports. It can occur in association with other injuries of the shoulder, or as a separate entity.

Signs. After injury to the bursa the player experiences some pain and limitation of shoulder movement the same evening. The next day he complains of diffuse pain and severe limitation of movement. When the bursa is palpated, as described on p. 103, pain is elicited.

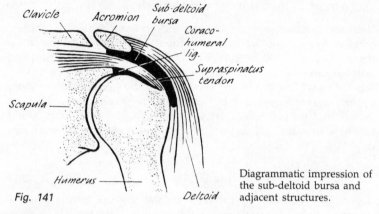

Fig. 141

Diagrammatic impression of the sub-deltoid bursa and adjacent structures.

Treatment

Movement of the shoulder irritates the inflamed bursa and sets up a chronic bursitis; this causes a gross limitation of movement.

The shoulder joint must be rested completely by supporting the arm and forearm in a triangular sling. The bursa is treated by daily applications of short-wave diathermy. The player is warned of the importance of keeping the shoulder still, and not taking the arm out of the sling for exercise.

If this treatment is followed conscientiously an acute bursitis will clear up within about 7 days.

Testing the injury. Before exercise is allowed the therapist should test the normal active movements of the shoulder (pp. 102–103). If movement is painless and the ranges are normal, the shoulder may be used freely and training can be resumed. If, however, pain is experienced on any of the tests treatment must be continued.

Strains and tears of the 'rotator cuff'

The term 'rotator cuff' is used to describe an important fibrous structure which surrounds the upper half of the head of the humerus. It is formed by the blending together of the tendons of the supraspinatus, infraspinatus, subscapularis and teres minor. These muscles are shown in Figs. 52 and 53, pp. 99 and 100.

Strains and partial or complete tears of the cuff tendons occur frequently; the supraspinatus tendon is the most commonly involved. (Fig. 142.)

Strain or partial tear of supraspinatus tendon

The supraspinatus tendon is injured by some sudden strain, e.g. fast bowling in cricket, a fall on the outstretched arm, or sudden strong abduction of the arm against the resistance of a heavy weight held in the hand.

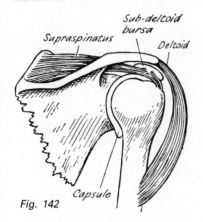

Sub-deltoid bursa

Supraspinatus

Deltoid

Capsule

Fig. 142

Diagram showing a partial tear of the supraspinatus tendon. Back view of right shoulder joint.

Signs of injury. The player complains of pain at the tip of the shoulder. When he raises the arm sideways-upward above his head pain occurs after the first 45° of movement; it diminishes when the arm reaches some 120°. The normal rhythm of shoulder abduction is disturbed; the player masks his inability to abduct the joint normally by shrugging up the shoulder girdle.

Treatment

The arm is generally rested in a triangular sling for 2 or 3 days. Pulsed short-wave or interferential therapy is used the day after injury, and is localized to the supraspinatus tendon. After the treatment has been given, shoulder exercises should be practised in the stooping position, as described in the section dealing with the after-treatment of a dislocated shoulder; the exercises must be progressed smoothly as indicated on p. 201.

Transverse frictions. From about the fourth day onwards transverse friction is applied very carefully to the injured tendon. The player is treated in lying, with the shoulder extended and inwardly rotated to keep the tendon on the stretch. The frictions are painful, and should only be given on alternate days.

Resuming training. With good treatment the injury usually clears up in about 3 to 4 weeks. Active tests of all shoulder movements (including range of movement) are carried out, as described on pp. 102–103; particular attention is paid to testing abduction and outward rotation. If the results are satisfactory, and the normal rhythm of shoulder abduction has been regained, training is resumed.

Part 6
Treatment of fractures and skin conditions

Chapter 17

Principles of fracture treatment

A fracture consists of the breaking of a bone. The bone may be fractured with or without displacement of the fragments; the fracture may also be accompanied by a dislocation of a neighbouring joint (fracture-dislocation).

A simple fracture is one in which the overlying skin is intact, while a compound fracture is one in which the fracture communicates with the skin surface by a wound. This does not necessarily mean that the broken bone ends are exposed or protruding through the wound. At the time of injury a compound fracture is always contaminated and potentially infected by clothing or dust.

Traumatic fractures. The force causing a fracture may consist of (1) Direct violence, e.g. an arm or leg is broken by a blow; (2) Indirect violence, as when the clavicle is fractured by a fall on the outstretched hand; and (3) Muscular action, as in a fracture of the patella due to a sudden contraction of the quadriceps muscle.

Fatigue or stress fractures. Fatigue fractures result from long-continued or oft-repeated stress; they have been likened to the fatigue fractures which sometimes occur in metal. They consist of hair-line cracks, and there is no displacement of the fragments.

'March' fracture occurs in the neck of the second metatarsal bone, most often in Army recruits. Fatigue fracture of the fibula occurs in long-distance runners at the weakest point of the bone at about the junction of the middle and lower thirds of the shaft. Fatigue fractures of the middle of the tibia occur in young healthy ballet dancers.

Treatment of fracture by plaster fixation

After correction of any displacement of the fragments the fracture is generally immobilized in a plaster-of-paris cast or a splint for several weeks; this allows union to occur and prevents re-displacement. During the period of immobilization certain changes take place in the

splinted tissues; some result from injury and some from fixation. The main changes are given below:
1. Wasting of the muscles.
2. Stiffening of the joints due to shortening of the ligaments and muscles, and the formation of adhesions.
3. Decalcification of bone (withdrawal of lime-salts).
4. Decreased tone in the walls of the blood and lymph vessels.

These changes can be minimized by regular exercise of (a) the muscles which are enclosed in the plaster cast or splint, and (b) the *free* joints and muscles in the vicinity of the fracture.

To demonstrate the types of exercises used a summary of the treatment of a fractured shaft of the tibia is given here. The fracture is immobilized by a plaster cast which extends from the webs of the toes to the groin; usually the knee is slightly flexed and the foot fixed at a right angle to the leg. The hip joint and toes are left free.

Exercises. When the plaster is dry the player practises static contractions of the quadriceps and hamstring muscles (pp. 45 and 143), and bending and stretching movements of the toes. The exercises are carried out on a 'little and often' basis. Generally the surgeon will also allow simple hip exercises, e.g. (a) Lying, raising the 'plaster' leg through 45°, and (b) Lying on the sound side, raising the leg sideways.

A few days later the player is usually allowed to exercise the muscles of the ankle and foot, a series of 'attempted' movements being used. For example, he attempts to bend and stretch the ankle and to turn the foot inwards and outwards, although the cast prevents any appreciable movement from taking place. These 'attempted' exercises should be performed smoothly and fairly slowly.

When weight-bearing on the injured limb is permitted a large leather over-shoe is worn over the foot-piece of the cast, and the player is encouraged to walk normally. Sticks or elbow crutches are used until he can stand and walk without difficulty.

Treatment when fracture has united

When the fracture has united and the plaster cast is removed physiotherapy is essential. The main aims of treatment consist of strengthening the weak muscles, mobilizing the stiff joints and training the player to use the injured part normally. In lower limb fractures this includes training in walking and treatment to disperse swelling or oedema.

To demonstrate the various forms of therapy a summary of the treatment of a fractured shaft of the tibia is given here.

Exercises. At first *non-weight-bearing* exercises are used to mobilize the knee, ankle and foot, and to strengthen the thigh and leg muscles. For example, half-lying on a massage couch (Fig. 61, p. 114): (a) Bending and stretching the knee within the limit of pain with the heel kept in contact with the couch top; (b) Bending and stretching the ankles alternately (Fig. 18, p. 56); (c) Circling each foot in turn, and (d) Slow controlled bending and stretching of each ankle in turn. Later, the exercises should be progressed to *assisted* weight-bearing movements, e.g. heel raising from standing, with the hands holding a chair back or a wall-bar (Fig. 11, p. 47), and heel raising and knee bending through 90° from the same starting position. Resisted exercises to strengthen the quadriceps and calf muscles should also be used. *See* Fig. 15, p. 49.

Massage. The leg often swells when the player starts to stand and walk, because of the decreased tone of the walls of the blood and lymph vessels. General massage of the thigh, leg and foot, with the limb elevated on pillows, is helpful. After the massage the leg should be supported by a crêpe bandage which must extend from the webs of the toes to just below the knee (Fig. 90, p. 131); sometimes it is also necessary to support the knee with a crêpe bandage (Fig. 96, p. 136).

Elevation of the limb. To counteract the swelling of the leg the player should be encouraged to elevate the limb several times a day, either by lying down on a couch with the limb raised on pillows, or resting the foot on a stool when sitting.

Walking training. Usually the player needs two sticks when he starts to walk without the cast. He must be taught to take even steps, and to use the knee and ankle joints properly; often he tends to hold them stiffly.

Chapter 18

Injuries and infections of the skin

Injuries and infections of the skin are a common occurrence in all forms of sport. Many of them are of a comparatively minor nature. Unless they are treated promptly and efficiently, however, they can give rise to troublesome symptoms which may well hold up a player's progress.

Some of the commoner forms of skin injuries and infections are discussed here, together with their treatment.

Injuries of the skin

Abrasions

Abrasions or 'brush burns' occur chiefly in body-contact sports, especially when the playing surface is hard. Small or large areas of the skin are scraped or rubbed away by friction; the parts of the body most affected are the areas where the bone lies close to the skin.

Treatment. Abrasions should be cleaned with an antiseptic lotion, such as Savlon; any dirt or grit in the wound must be removed carefully. The player is then referred to the club doctor, because it is usual to give an injection of anti-tetanus serum after any injury where the skin has been broken and there is a possibility that the wound has been infected by contact with the ground, either in a direct or indirect manner. If the doctor is not available the player must be sent to the nearest hospital.

The trainer or the therapist should keep a written record of the date of the injection, together with details of the player's reaction to the serum.

Dressings. Small abrasions do not usually require dressings. They are often painted with gentian violet.

Large abrasions are covered with white sterile lint which has been either saturated with acriflavine lotion or covered with one of the antiseptic creams, e.g. Savlon or Cetavlex. The lint is held in place by narrow strips of zinc oxide plaster. It is most important that the dressing is not completely covered by strapping; if this is done the air cannot reach the wound and it becomes soggy and healing is delayed.

The wounds should be examined daily, and the dressings renewed under aseptic conditions. Treatment by infra-red radiation is often helpful in healing the larger abrasions; a mild heat is used for about 15 to 20 minutes each day.

Delayed healing. Abrasions which do not heal satisfactorily should be seen by the doctor; he may advise the use of penicillin nonad tulle dressings. If the abrasion becomes infected the doctor must also be informed; signs of infection are redness, pain and swelling of the nearby lymph glands.

Blisters

Blisters of the hands and feet are a fairly common occurrence at the start of the playing season. They should be treated as soon as possible.

The blister and the adjacent area of skin are swabbed with an anti-septic lotion (e.g. Savlon or Cetavlex); one side of the blister is then pricked with a needle which has been previously sterilized by being held in a spirit flame for a few moments or boiled for about 6 minutes. A piece of sterile gauze or lint is then placed over the blister, and gentle pressure applied to squeeze out the fluid. The skin is then swabbed again with antiseptic lotion, and collodion applied; this is followed by a dry sterile dressing.

Prevention of blisters. At the beginning of training it is a wise precaution to toughen the skin by the regular use of methylated spirit or alum powder.

Lacerations

Lacerations consist of irregular tears of the skin and superficial tissues combined with bruising. They are cleaned with an antiseptic lotion and covered with sterile dressings. Deep lacerations need to be stit-ched, and must be dealt with by the club doctor; if he is not available the player must be sent to hospital. The stitches are usually taken out after about 7 days. Up to this time the injured part is kept covered with a dry sterile dressing.

Anti-tetanus serum. An injection of anti-tetanus serum is given as a routine procedure. *See* Treatment of abrasions, p. 212.

Infections of the skin

'Athlete's foot', 'toe-rot' or tinea pedis

This is not only an extremely common skin condition, but often a difficult one to cure completely. The skin between the clefts of the toes or on the sole of the foot becomes infected by a vegetable fungus, the *trichophyton*. At first the condition is often unrecognized. Later there is some degree of itching; the skin between the toes thickens and becomes white and sodden-looking; coarse scales and horny thickenings occur on the sole. Infection is spread by the common use of baths, showers, bath mats and borrowed socks and shoes.

Prevention of infection. Before entering and on leaving the shower or bathroom the players should step into a foot-bath containing an antiseptic solution, e.g. 10 per cent Dettol. They must dry their feet thoroughly, particularly in between the toes, and report at once to the trainer or the therapist if they develop any skin irritation or eruptions. Towels and socks used by infected players must be kept apart from the other players' kit. The towels should be boiled after each training session; the socks should be soaked in a 10 per cent solution of Dettol for about 20 minutes, and then washed thoroughly.

Treatment. The regular and persistent use of an anti-fungoid ointment and powder (e.g. Mycil or Tineafax) will generally clear up the condition, although it may tend to recur from time to time. The ointment is rubbed into the affected areas of the skin at night before going to bed and in the morning before putting on the socks. It is helpful if the feet are washed and dried thoroughly before the ointment is applied. During the day two or three applications of powder are used.

Treatment may have to be continued for several weeks or even months in severe cases.

Griseofulvin. This is an antibiotic which is sometimes used in the treatment of 'Athlete's foot' and other fungus conditions of the skin. It is taken by mouth in the form of tablets, and is thought to act by endowing the skin cells with the power to resist fungi completely. The drug is available only on the prescription of a doctor, and is used over a period of several weeks.

Boils or furuncles

A boil is caused by a staphyloccocal infection of a hair follicle or a sweat gland. Two factors contribute to the development of boils: a general lowered resistance and a local irritation – pressure, friction or scratching.

Treatment. Penicillin therapy is often prescribed by the doctor. Short-wave diathermy is also extremely useful, provided that a *mild* heating only is used. The gentle heat improves the circulation through the affected area of the skin without increasing the activity of the bacteria. By improving the circulation more white blood corpuscles are brought to the area to separate the central core of pus from the healthy tissues and to promote healing.

Two 10-minute sessions of short-wave diathermy are given each day before and after the boil discharges. When the boil is discharging it should be cleaned under aseptic conditions before treatment is given. Between treatments it should be kept covered by a dressing of sterile gauze which is held in place by one or two narrow strips of zinc oxide plaster.

Cellulitis

Cellulitis is a spreading bacterial infection of the tissues which lie immediately under the skin. It gives rise to a boggy, tender, red swelling of the tissues, which is associated with a severe throbbing pain and a rise of temperature. The infection may originate from a boil or a puncture wound of the skin.

The condition is mentioned here because it is important that the trainer should be able to recognize it. When cellulitis occurs the player must be referred at once to the doctor.

'Dhobie itch' or tinea cruris

This is a similar condition to 'Athlete's foot', but the fungus infects the skin of the groin and the fold between the buttocks; sometimes it spreads to the armpits. The condition can be caught from a W.C. seat.

Prevention and treatment. On the lines suggested for 'Athlete's foot' (p. 214). The underclothes of the infected player should be changed each day; before being washed they should be either boiled or soaked for 20 minutes in a 10 per cent solution of Dettol.

Lymphangitis

After a puncture wound of the skin the lymphatic vessels of the area sometimes become infected. The infection spreads rapidly up the lymphatics to the nearest lymphatic glands, which generally succeed in limiting it. The inflamed lymphatics stand out as tender red cords and the glands are swollen, hard and painful.

If lymphangitis is suspected the player must be referred at once to the doctor. Delay in obtaining medical advice may lead to the infection spreading to the main blood stream.

Part 7

First-aid and prevention of injury

Part 3

First aid and prevention of injuries

Chapter 19
First-aid on the field or track

First-aid calls for considerable experience and skill on the part of the trainer or therapist. He must not only be efficient at giving immediate treatment, but must be capable of assessing the injury and determining whether or not the player should be allowed to continue in the game or event.

Severe injuries, such as dislocations and fractures, present him with fewer *immediate* problems than the less severe injuries; first-aid is applied on the field or track, and the player removed for examination by the club doctor. In dealing with the less severe injuries, such as sprains, muscle tears and bruises, the trainer's decision is influenced by the degree of pain felt by the player and the amount of difficulty he experiences in moving the injured part.

Four rules to be observed by the trainer are given here:

1. When in doubt remove the player for examination by the doctor.
2. Ask the player how the injury occurred, e.g. Was it the result of a direct blow or a twist?
3. When the trunk or lower extremity is injured the player must not be allowed to stand before examination.
4. The injured part must not be moved passively or manipulated before examination. Passive movement or manipulation can convert a minor injury into a major one.

Common injuries and their first-aid treatment

Concussion

This condition is a temporary loss of consciousness due to a blow on the head. The loss of consciousness is caused by the violent movement of the head, which disturbs the normal functioning of the brain. The player may lose consciousness for a few seconds or minutes, or for a much longer period; this may vary from one or two hours to a day or more.

If the head injury is severe there may be a fracture of one of the bones of the skull, with associated damage to the blood vessels. This type of injury can have fatal results.

When the player recovers consciousness he may be dull and listless and not fully aware of his surroundings. On other occasions the player's general reactions are grossly exaggerated. There is always a loss of memory after concussion, and the actual blow is never clearly remembered.

First-aid. When the player is unconscious for only a few seconds the trainer must be absolutely certain that he has fully recovered before allowing him to continue in the game or event. If the player has been unconscious for a few minutes, the trainer is well advised to refer the player to the doctor, and not to take the responsibility upon himself.

Recovery position. An unconscious player or athlete should always be removed from the field or track on a stretcher *lying on his side* with the knee of the uppermost side drawn up to act as a prop for the lower part of the body, and the arm of the same side bent at the elbow to prop up the upper part. His head should be turned to the same side and rested on a *thin* towel or handkerchief, so that any vomit can drain from his mouth if he is sick.

He must not be left lying on his back. This is vitally important from the point of view of maintaining a clear airway, which can easily become blocked by vomit or secretions, or the tongue dropping backwards. Blocking of the airway may lead to the brain being deprived of oxygen. Irretrievable damage may result.

In assessing the player after a head injury the trainer must concentrate on the following points:
1. Is there any bleeding from the eyes, ears or nose?
2. Are the eyes reacting normally to light?
3. Is the player mentally dull or excitable?

If the trainer is in any doubt about any of these points the player must be removed from the field or track.

Stimulants should never be given after concussion. A 24-hour rest is advisable if the player has not been allowed to continue in the game or event; members of his family should be instructed to call a doctor at once if his behaviour changes and becomes different from normal.

Contusions or bruises

A contusion is the result of a kick or direct contact with another player, or a heavy fall on a hard surface. Usually the skin is not broken, but some degree of bleeding occurs within the superficial tissues because of damage to the small blood vessels; the affected part tends to stiffen, mainly because of pain and muscle spasm.

Most players will be allowed to continue with the game or event.

An attempt should be made to localize the bleeding by strapping the part with elastoplast over a sponge-rubber or felt pad.

Cramp

A cramp is a sustained and extremely painful contraction of one or more muscle groups. The mechanism of the condition is not fully understood, but it may be due to some upset of the nervous control of the muscle fibres, or to an impaired circulation. Cramp frequently occurs when a muscle group has been subjected to intensive training, or is used in a sudden vigorous manner.

First-aid. The affected muscles should be put on the stretch (either by the trainer or the player) and maintained in this position until the spasm subsides. For example, in dealing with cramp of the calf muscles the trainer can passively dorsiflex the ankle to the full extent, with the knee straight, or the player can take up a lunge position.

A possible cause of cramp in football players is their practice of keeping up their stockings with strips of bandage or bootlaces, which are tied tightly round the legs. The trainer should insist on the use of elastic garters.

A player who is frequently troubled by cramp should be referred to the club doctor.

Cuts and abrasions

Superficial cuts are first cleaned with an antiseptic lotion, such as Savlon; collodion is then applied, and the part covered with a sterile dressing. Deep cuts may need stitching; they should be cleaned, and the player referred as soon as possible to the club doctor.

Abrasions are treated in the same way as superficial cuts, but acriflavine is used instead of collodion.

Dressings for the limbs are best fastened in position by encircling straps of elastoplast; small dressings on the face and trunk may be fastened by strips of zinc oxide strapping.

Anti-tetanus serum injection. After the game or event the trainer should consult the club doctor about the advisability of an anti-tetanus serum injection. If this is given the trainer should keep a written record.

Fractures and dislocations

No attempt should be made by the trainer to reduce a fracture or dislocation. He should immobilize the injured part as soon as possible, and supervise the removal of the player to hospital. Stimulants or drinks of any kind are prohibited, because the player may be given a general anaesthetic when he is treated at the hospital.

Torn semilunar cartilage

When one of the semilunar cartilages is torn the knee sometimes 'locks' in about 30° of flexion. The trainer should not attempt to straighten the joint, but should ask the club doctor to see the player. If the doctor is not available the player should be sent to hospital at once. It is important that a medical man should see the player with the knee 'locked', so that a diagnosis of torn cartilage may be established. If the trainer manipulates the knee and reduces the displaced cartilage valuable clinical evidence is lost.

Once the cartilage is torn it must be removed by the surgeon. Often there is a considerable delay between the time of injury and the operation, because the player is not seen with the knee 'locked', and the surgeon has insufficient evidence of a cartilage tear.

Injuries of testicles and scrotum

Bruising of the testes and scrotum occurs when they are struck by a ball or involved in direct body contact. The injury is extremely painful and incapacitating. Sometimes the pain passes off fairly quickly and treatment is not required; on other occasions pain and spasm are prolonged and treatment is essential.

The player should be removed from the field or track. A sponge or towel should be soaked in hot water, squeezed out, and applied to the scrotum; the player should be encouraged to pass urine. The relief of pain produced by this treatment is often dramatic. If the player passes blood in the urine, medical advice should be sought before he is allowed to return to the field or track.

The trainer should make a practice of including a small vacuum flask of hot water in his first-aid box, so that he can deal promptly with injuries of this type.

Rib injuries

The ribs and their muscles are often bruised; sometimes the ribs and the sternum (breast-bone) are fractured.

Fracture. The trainer palpates the injured area of the chest carefully; abnormal movement or grating indicates that one or more of the ribs is fractured.

The player should be removed from the field or track, and strapping applied round the chest at the level of the injury. Two or three parallel turns of 2½ in. elastoplast are used; as they are applied the player should breathe out as much as possible.

After being strapped the player is sent to hospital. It is dangerous to allow him to continue with the game or event because the broken ends of the rib might puncture the covering of the lung or the lung tissue. This could result in serious complications.

Bruising. The player is instructed to breathe out, and the chest is strapped firmly as described above. The player may then return to the field or track.

Muscle and tendon tears

A muscle, its tendon or its sheath can be torn by a vigorous contraction or some sudden incoordinated movement. The injury varies from a tearing of a few fibres to a complete rupture of the structure involved, and is always associated with some degree of pain and loss of function. A common site of injury is the junction of the muscle with its tendon.

Minor tears. The injured part is strapped firmly with elastoplast over a pad of felt or sponge rubber. The player is then allowed to continue in the game or event.

Major tears. The player is removed from the field or track and referred to the club doctor.

Sprains

A sprain consists of a tearing of some of the fibres of a ligament (*see* p. 112). When a minor sprain occurs the player can usually continue in the game or event if the joint is bandaged or strapped firmly.

Some football trainers believe that it is better not to remove the player's boot after a minor sprain of the ankle. They advocate pouring cold water or spirit into the boot top, and then applying elastoplast over the boot. This is *not* a procedure to follow; the degree of support afforded is inadequate.

In rugby football the ligaments of the fingers are often sprained. Splintage can be provided by strapping the adjacent sound finger to the injured one (p. 186); zinc oxide plaster is used.

Severe sprains. Players with severe sprains of the ligaments should be removed from the field or track and referred to the club doctor. Often these injuries are associated with fractures.

The 'winded' player

In body-contact sports the player is often 'winded' as a result of a blow in the region of the solar plexus. The blow produces a momentary paralysis of the diaphragm and spasm of the abdominal muscles; respiration is impaired.

The trainer must reassure the player; he applies a cold sponge to the nape of the neck, and allows him to remain in whatever position he finds most comfortable. Some trainers encourage the player to stand up, and then proceed to move his head and trunk up and down in 'pump-handle' style. This does no good, and may be very dangerous, because the condition may not be a straightforward one; other structures may be injured – kidneys, spine or ribs.

Generally the player recovers quickly after being 'winded'. If he recovers slowly, and seems shocked and restless, he should be removed from the field or track; the trainer should seek medical advice.

Heart attack and heart failure – emergency measures

During athletic activities the sportsman may suffer a heart attack or, if he is very unfortunate, a heart failure, or complete arrest of cardiac function (technically known as cardiac arrest).

The main symptoms of a heart attack consist of pain over the chest, possibly radiating down the left arm. They are associated with considerable physical distress and profuse sweating.

In heart failure the sportsman collapses, lapsing into unconsciousness. He turns a blue-grey colour, the pupils of the eyes dilate, and there is no pulse at neck or wrist.

First-aid measures. In heart failure resuscitation procedures must be applied immediately, as taught in standard first-aid manuals and classes.

In a heart attack it is essential to position the sportsman correctly. Often this is mismanaged and he is placed flat on his back on the ground, well-intentioned helpers believing that this will relieve strain on the heart. The reverse is true, of course. It is essential that the sportsman should be placed in a *supported sitting position, with hips and knees flexed*, to relax off the abdominal wall and so assist diaphragmatic breathing.

Heat stroke and heat exhaustion

Many sports are now played in a variety of climatic extremes. It is of the greatest importance that the symptoms of heat stroke and heat exhaustion should be recognized immediately, and prompt action taken to counteract the conditions.

Heat stroke. Heat stroke can occur almost without warning, and is due to a breakdown of the normal sweating process which regulates the body temperature. The warning signs consist of a high temperature (40°C or 104°F) and rapid pulse; these are associated with a hot, dry skin and noisy breathing. Headache, dizziness and restlessness may accompany these symptoms. They may lead on to mental confusion and unconsciousness.

Treatment. Correct first-aid measures must be applied immediately. The sportsman should be placed in a back-lying position and effective cooling procedures instituted – sponging down the body (which should be stripped) with cold water, or applying cold compresses and packs, plus fanning from above. An alternative measure consists of wrapping the sportsman in a cold wet sheet, and keeping it wet until his temperature has fallen to 38°C (100°F).

If a doctor is available he should be contacted immediately. Failing this, the sportsman should be sent to hospital.

Heat exhaustion. Unlike heat stroke the onset of this condition is slow. The sportsman sweats excessively and loses very large amounts of water and salt. He is restless and plainly exhausted, with a pale cold face, clammy with sweat, although his body temperature does not vary a great deal from normal. Pulse and respiration are rapid, and muscular cramps may occur due to loss of salt.

Treatment. The sportsman should be moved immediately to a cool place. If he is conscious he should be given a drink of cold water, to which common salt has been added (half a teaspoonful to a pint of water). If a doctor is available he should be notified at once.

Chapter 20

Prevention of injury

Training increases body endurance, strength, speed and efficiency. Players who have not trained to their full capacity are liable to sustain injuries during play, because fatigue or imperfect coordination lead to faulty movements.

Training may be divided into (1) Endurance training, (2) Strength or power training, and (3) Skill training. These are interrelated, and it is often possible to carry them out simultaneously.

Training

Endurance training aims at developing the efficiency of the heart and lungs, so that the blood and oxygen supply to the working muscles is increased. This facilitates the functioning of the muscles and reduces fatigue.

The training consists of (1) General rhythmical exercises, (2) Running and skipping, (3) Minor team games, (4) Circuit training, and (5) High repetition lifts with low weights. It should also include the types of movements which are related to specific forms of sport, e.g. starting, stopping and direction-changing movements would feature in the endurance training programme of a rugby, hockey or soccer player.

Strength or power training is necessary to prepare the player for the 'expulsive effort', e.g. moving quickly into the open space or racing for a 'loose ball'.

Power training includes (1) Strengthening exercises, (2) Sprinting, and (3) Low repetition lifts with heavy weights. All parts of the body should be exercised, and it is most important that the upper extremity should not be neglected. Press-ups, pull-ups, hand-stand press-ups, weight-and-pulley exercises, and activities such as 'Wrist wrestle' are particularly useful.

Proof of the importance of developing the muscles of the upper extremity can be seen when one looks at the international sprinter; the arms and shoulder-girdle are developed in a similar degree to the lower limbs.

Skill training. Skill is a vital factor in reducing the incidence of injury, and the player must spend many hours in practising the individual skills of his game. For example, the tennis player should practise the service, smash, forehand and backhand strokes, and be able to recover quickly; the soccer player should practise trapping, dribbling, swerving, turning, kicking the moving ball, timing the tackle, quick direction changing and heading; he must be able to use each foot with equal skill, and swerve or turn to left or right with ease.

Training and staleness

Players often ask: How much training is necessary? The answer is simple: the maximum amount in relation to the game or event. Correct training cannot reduce the efficiency of any player, and it does not cause staleness, as is sometimes thought.

Staleness is the bogey of all trainers and players. The player feels that his muscles are 'heavy', and his performance loses its edge; often he sums this up by saying that he seems to have no 'snap' in his body.

Staleness is probably caused by psychological factors, although it is not always easy to find the exact source of the trouble. Some factors which are worth considering in this respect are given below:
1. Has the training routine become monotonous? How often has it been varied?
2. Is the player happy at home? Does he have regular and sound meals?
3. Is the player completely fit? Has he contracted an illness which has not been diagnosed?
4. Has the player an injury which he is trying to hide?
5. Is the player mentally and physically equipped for the game or event? Is he of the 'worrying' type?
6. Is there complete harmony among the players? Is the team losing more matches than it is winning?
7. Is the player unpopular with a section of the crowd?

Resuming training after injury

Testing for fitness. Before an injured player is allowed to resume training the damaged structures must be thoroughly tested. This involves both specific tests of ligaments and muscles (pp. 82–103) and functional tests, as described on p. 81.

If a ligament has been injured the structures are put on the stretch by passive movements; pain at the beginning or middle part of the movement indicates that further treatment is necessary, and training cannot be resumed. If pain is not experienced, or is apparent only when the structures are *fully* stretched, training can be resumed and treatment discontinued.

When a muscle or tendon has been injured the structures are put through a full range of active or resisted movement. Absence of pain (or slight pain on the final degrees of resisted movement) indicates that treatment can be discontinued and training started.

Strapping. When training is resumed the injured structures should be supported by some form of strapping, such as zinc oxide plaster, elastoplast, or a combination of both forms of strapping. The strapping must be applied carefully, without folds or creases; this is particularly important after injuries of the ankle and foot. An indifferently applied ankle or foot support can easily cause soreness or blistering of the skin. To protect the part the player automatically holds his foot in a different position from normal; this alters the coordination of the part and may result in injury.

Graduated training. At first training should be relatively light. It should be increased gradually until finally the player is practising all the skills and basic movements of the game.

Examining the injury. The injured part should be examined the day after training to check for any recurrence of injury; this practice should be continued over several training sessions. Whenever possible the injured structures should be compared with the corresponding sound tissues. Points to look out for on examination are: swelling, pain on palpation and movement, and undue warmth at the site of injury.

Care of the feet

The feet form the springboard of many of the movements which are made by the body in sport. A small foot defect such as a blister, ingrowing toe nail or corn can interfere with the normal function of the foot and cause an injury to the lower limb or spine.

Most players pay considerable attention to the fit of their shoes or boots, but give little or no thought to the fit of their socks or stockings. Tight socks interfere with the growth of the nails and the function of the toes; darns may cause corns, and holes give rise to blisters.

Testing for functional fitness after injury

When the training programme starts it should not only be progressive and functional in nature, but include all the physical situations and stresses required of the player or athlete. The successful completion of such a training programme enables him to return with confidence to his game or event.

Training sessions should begin with extensibility exercises and progress to preparatory and warming-up activities. The following programme is suitable for the soccer player.

Jogging
1. Jog 55 yards, walk 55 yards. Repeat 4 times.
2. Jog 110 yards, walk 110 yards. Repeat 4 times.
3. Jog 55 yards, walk 55 yards. Repeat 4 times.

Walking
4. Walking; arms circling.
5. Walking; trunk turning to left and right with arms swinging round the body.

Jogging
6. Jogging; touch right foot with right hand, then left foot with left hand.
7. Jogging; single high knee raising (left and then right).

The exercises should now be carried out at a quicker pace.

Running
8. Running; arms circling.
9. Running; on command turn sideways to left and then to right.
10. Running; check on left foot and then on right foot.
11. Running; high jump, arms reaching to the sky.
12. Running; jumping high to head an imaginary football.
13. Running; knee raise and turn hip outward, single and then alternate.
14. Running; left leg kicking forward, right leg kicking forward.
15. Running; turn, run backward – turn – run forward.
16. Running; jumping to head an imaginary football: to left and then to right.
17. Running forward; turn and kick left, then right (as high as possible).
18. Running at speed; on command touch ground on left, then ground on right.

Jogging
19. Jogging; on command go off in various directions at speed.
20. Jogging; sprint, then high jump with arms reaching to the sky.
21. Jogging; then 25-yard sprint, then 50-yard sprint.
22. Jogging; running, changing direction every 5 or 10 yards.

Deep breathing should be encouraged between each activity.

Further preparation

Before the player returns to a competitive game the trainer must be convinced that he is capable of meeting the physical demands which will be required of him. A game of soccer requires variations in speed from jogging to sprinting in various directions, sudden stops and quick changes in direction.

During running the trainer must ensure that the player's paces are even and that each heel is raised behind to the same level. The player should be required to travel at varying speeds *with a football* – sprinting, dribbling, interpassing at speed, tackling and shooting.

It is essential to test the player for all the requirements of a competitive game of soccer. These requirements can be summarised as: speed, agility, skill, strength, flexibility, endurance, reaction, balance and confidence.

It is worth noting that during a recent first-division English football league match a well-known striker travelled the following distances:
Trotting and medium running, 3,813 yards
Fast running and sprinting, 1,247 yards
Running sideways, 130 yards
Walking forward, 1,682 yards
Walking backward, 130 yards
Deliberate change of direction, 453 times
In possession of the ball, 56 times

Index

233